PRAISE FOR DOLORE
THERAPEUTIC 1

"The association between touch and healing is ancient and worldwide. Skilled hands are among the physician's most important diagnostic and therapeutic tools. The importance of touch in medicine has been amply demonstrated . . . in our own time, by nurse/healer Dolores Krieger."
—*The Journal of the American Medical Association*

"A dynamo of a nurse and teacher, [Dolores Krieger] has transformed the practice of laying on of hands into a healing therapy. She has spent years stripping away the aura of mystique, superstition, and suspicion that has confined healing to a select group and opened it up to all."
—*East West/Natural Health*

"Laying on of hands gains new respect!"   —*The New York Times*

"Therapeutic Touch has the support of its enthusiasts because their experience indicates that it works. It's a learned procedure whose practitioners report good results."   —*Omni*

"There is a quiet revolution taking place in American medicine. The goal: to unite the high-tech wizardry of Western medical approaches with the low-tech, individualized attention of Eastern health care. This union . . . would create a system as strong on prevention as it is on intervention. Under Dr. Krieger's guidance the technique of therapeutic Touch has quietiy crept in hospital wards throughout the world."
—*Self Magazine*

"Dolores Krieger . . . is the undisputed doyenne of the Therapeutic Touch movement."   —*New Age Journal*

"One of the newest breakthroughs in medicine is as old as mankind—the ability to heal through touch . . . now scientists are beginning to understand the extraordinary ability of touch to help us heal our physical and emotional pain."   —*Ladies' Home Journal*

"Dolores Krieger is almost singlehandedly responsible for the spread of this modern version of the old laying-on-of-hands technique . . . it has become impossible to talk about Therapeutic Touch without talking about Dr. Krieger . . . the stuff of which miracles are made."
                              —*McCall's*

"Dr. Krieger 's own work with babies is particularly impressive."
                              —*American Baby*

"Dr. Dolores Krieger is turning faith healing into a recognized science. . . . Due in no small part to [her] efforts, [Therapeutic Touch] is being taught as a serious science to hundreds of health professionals across the country and is even being used in hospitals."   —*New York Magazine*

"Therapeutic Touch, first describe by Krieger in 1975 as an act of healing or helping that is akin to the ancient practice of laying on of hands . . . goes beyond placebo and involves an undefined but learnable method of human-energy balancing. In a world of expensive tools and high technology, human touch has been rediscoved as a valuable therapeutic method with dramatic implications."
                              —*American Journal of Nursing*

"Dr. Dolores Kreiger is creating a potential tidal wave in modern medicine, and her work is very important in restoring the heart and soul of healing. Importantly, she has gone *through* science, not around it, in her work with Therapeutic Touch. I have greatly admired her courage and vision for years. It is time for everyone to become aware of her magnificent discoveries."
                              —Larry Dossey, M.D., *author of Space, Time & Medicine*
                              and *Recovering the Soul*

THERAPEUTIC
TOUCH

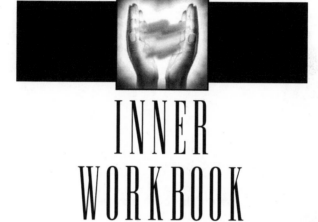

INNER
WORKBOOK

VENTURES IN TRANSPERSONAL HEALING

Dolores Krieger, Ph.D., R.N.

Foreword by
Jeanne Achterberg, Ph.D.

BEAR & COMPANY
PUBLISHING
SANTA FE, NEW MEXICO

LIBRARY OF CONGRESS CATALOGING-IN-PUBLICATION

Krieger, Dolores.
    Therapeutic touch inner workbook : ventures in transpersonal
healing / Dolores Krieger.
        p.   cm.
    Includes bibliographical references and index.
    ISBN 978-1-879181-39-7
    1. Touch–Therapeutic use. 2. Mental healing. 3. Vital force–
Therapeutic use. I. Title
RZ999.K754 1996
615.8'52–dc20   96-26342
                                                           CIP

Bear & Company, Inc.
Santa Fe, NM 87504-2860

Cover illustration: James Finnell
Cover and interior design: Melinda Belter
Text illustrations: Patricia Stewart
Editing: Gerry Clow, Sarah Zarbock, Sonya Moore
Printed in the United States of America by Lake Book Manufacturing

9 8 7 6 5 4

To Fritz, who taught me

that life is a game (Skt., *lilâ*),

And Dora,

who taught me to laugh.

CONTENTS

ILLUSTRATIONS & TABLES

FOREWORD

When Dee Krieger called and asked if I would write the foreword to her new book, I was humbly awed and responded very quickly that I could refuse her nothing. Her vision has advanced the world of health care beyond measure. The technique, Therapeutic Touch, is far more than a protocol for aiding and abetting the progress of illness; it is also a way of regarding the condition of humanity that has been too long absent in modern medicine. And even more, her work provides an exceptional experience for the practitioners—one that examines and honors the true nature of the healer. There is still another agenda in Dee's work, planned or unplanned: as a nurse, she has served as a pathfinder for a new dimension in her profession that has had reverberations all over the world. Because of her unique status at New York University, she has inspired research as well as clinical applications for the nursing profession.

My first experience with Dee's work was around 1978 when I participated in one of the early conferences sponsored by the Nurse Healer's Cooperative in New York City. At the very traditional medical school where I served as a faculty member, Therapeutic Touch was not exactly a household word, and I knew nothing of its conceptual basis. What I did know, as I looked out onto the audience of several hundred people at Dee's conference, was that there was an ineffable quality in their demeanour that was highly unusual. And I knew immediately that if I was ever in need of help or healing, I wanted someone to be with me through crisis with those characteristics—whatever they were.

In this book, Dee describes the phenomenological experience of one who practices Therapeutic Touch. She describes those aspects of consciousness of the healer that so enchanted and puzzled me years ago. The centering of oneself in order to be fully present with the person seeking healing and the nature of focusing attention with intentionality may well be at the core of all healing interventions, with all other tools and skills and medicaments merely the observed vehicle for transmission of the healing itself.

The power of human interconnectedness is a stunning force. We are by no means benign in one another's presence. We are made well and sick by our relationships with others. A vast amount of research is being accumulated which suggests (what earlier cultures absolutely knew) that invisible bonds connect us in a giant cosmic web. Our thoughts and emotions appear to travel with no regard to time or space and dance through the dreams and waking ideation and even the physical bodies of others. Our task is now to bring this fact to consciousness, and to stay awake and aware of the profoundly sacred nature of human relationship. Nowhere is this charge more important than in the world of health care. The work that Dee describes *is* a pure act of bringing forth the role of the relationship between two or more individuals in the healing forum.

This book is an inner workbook as its title suggests, and is full of rich experiential offerings. It is an inner workbook of still another sort: it challenges the intellect by contextualizing the information in research, and in ancient and enduring systems of thought found in many spiritual or esoteric traditions. The concept of energy, for instance, is one of the most controversial (and therefore exciting) areas in alternative (or complementary) health practices, certainly including Therapeutic Touch. In order to grasp its nature, it is vital to consider it from a basic research perspective, from personal experience, and from the golden stream of enduring wisdom, as Dee has done.

The work that is described so lucidly in these pages will change lives. It has mine.

Jeanne Achterberg, Ph.D., is the senior editor of *Alternative Therapies in Health and Medicine*, author of *Imagery in Healing* and *Woman as Healer*, co-author of *Rituals in Healing*, and executive faculty member, Saybrook Institute, San Francisco.

PREFACE & ACKNOWLEDGMENTS

The *Therapeutic Touch Inner Workbook* is a personal exploration of the healing act as perceived through the practice of Therapeutic Touch. This "inner work" book focuses on this extended range of experience, assuming that the reader is cognizant of previous books on Therapeutic Touch and has put that information into practice.[1]

In Therapeutic Touch as in the martial arts, persons playing the role of healer have to be more than masters of techniques; they must be masters of themselves. Techniques, in fact, form the less important aspect of Therapeutic Touch. The mastery of self is prompted by a unique contribution of Therapeutic Touch, in which the therapist centers her or his consciousness at the beginning of the Therapeutic Touch engagement. However, unlike other healing modalities that use their techniques in series, the Therapeutic Touch processes involve working in parallel; that is, the therapist remains on center throughout the Therapeutic Touch interaction, even while engaging in the integral healing techniques of the Therapeutic Touch process.

It is undeniably this continued sensitivity to the higher orders of the inner self that empowers Therapeutic Touch. In the process, this act of interiority indelibly marks the inner life of the individual so engaged. The subtle transformation presents opportunities for the perceptive therapist to actualize potential abilities while in the service of compassionate regard for those in need. This personal arena of the Therapeutic Touch engagement has been little studied, where the profound power of compassion reveals itself to a pragmatic society that is largely unaware of the incredible strengths of the inner self.

The *Therapeutic Touch Inner Workbook* is an attempt toward a clearer understanding of the inner reach of the healing moment. It examines the

---

[1]For example, D. Krieger, *Accepting Your Power to Heal: The Personal Practice of Therapeutic Touch.* (Santa Fe: Bear & Co., 1993); D. Krieger, *Therapeutic Touch: How to Use Your Hands to Help or to Heal.* (New York: Simon and Schuster, Prentice-Hall Press, 1979).

inner workplace of the healer through creative imagery, metaphor, analogy, and most importantly, the experience of specific exercises designed to challenge the well-practiced, thoughtful therapist. Dialogues with the reader are interspersed throughout in which implications of fundamental knowledge of the Therapeutic Touch experience are considered. One goal of the book is to deepen the conscious awareness of the journey undertaken by the therapist who would be healer. Its goal is also to strengthen the effectiveness of the teaching and practice of Therapeutic Touch; to suggest creative and satisfying questions for future research; and to develop the theory underlying Therapeutic Touch as a healing practice and as a singular avenue for personal growth.

● ● ●

The *Therapeutic Touch Inner Workbook* is a work whose insights evolved over the past six or seven years; however, it was only recently that I understood its message. It came about in this way: frequently in the midst of a lecture or class, I would be about to lauch into information on the deeper reaches of Therapeutic Touch when the thought would trigger a strong sense of caution. Verbalized, it went something like this: "Slow down, Krieger. Give them (the students) the permission for their own Therapeutic Touch practices to elicit these thoughts for themselves. Give them the opportunity to think these ideas through. Don't crowd, don't push, give them time to make the experience their own."

It was only about two years ago that I awoke to the stunning AH-HA! that it was not "them;" it was *me*. It was I who had to recognize and understand the deeper content of the Therapeutic Touch experience well enough to accurately teach it within its own appropriate context. This challenge gave me permission to study in-depth the dynamics of this intimate healer-healee interaction; to test the emerging ideas in subsequent classes and workshops; and to analyze the results and write my findings in the present manuscript. The writing of the manuscript involved allowing rigorous analysis and creative freedom to live side by side within me. It resulted in a personally confrontational, deeply satisfying, and thrilling engagement. The developing mood of it I associate with other in-depth meditative experiences; and, as with those meditative experiences, I sensed in the resultant insights a significant stretching of the boundaries of my own little world as well.

Looking back at that journey, I realized that I am personally deeply indebted to several people. Of critical importance to the present work is F.L. Kunz, who taught me how to assemble large amounts of related facts, search out the underlying principles that bound them together, and derive from these principles appropriate concepts that would integrate and clarify the many ideas latent in the initial mass of information.

From this personal perspective, I also acknowledge Emily B. Sellon, who encouraged me since early in my searches of "the healing ways" to seek out my own interpretation of life and living but, as should opinion, "hold it in your hand, but lightly."

Thirdly, but most importantly, I acknowledge Dora Kunz, who mentored, inspired, and supported me, and did, indeed, teach me to laugh, most especially at my own rather strange absurdities. Over the past quarter-century this relationship has been the source of unqualified delight and unreserved pride to have developed with her Therapeutic Touch.

On the professional front, it gives me particular pleasure to acknowledge Jeanne Achterberg, Ph.D., whose keen grasp of healing as a compassionate enactment which naturally couples mind and emotions in quest of the living harmonic we call health has lead the way to unique interpretations of the interior processes by which that state is attained. Her several researches, particularly in reference to persons with cancer, clearly demonstrates the unexpected extent to which the mysteries of the unconscious can engage themselves in the cause of self-healing. She stands as model of excellence in quest and in deed for many of us in these last days "between parentheses," and I am very proud that she has written the foreword to this book.

I would like also to acknowledge the editorial support of Barbara and Gerry Clow, who taught me the value of a well-placed comma, the power of a turn of phrase, and the "rightness" of a period—whose time had come!

I appreciate the special monitoring by Sarah F. Zarbock of the technical aspects of the book that concern physiological correlates, and I value equally Patricia Stewart's artistry in translating inarticulate ideas into illustrative graphic form. Jody Winters, publicist at Bear & Company, never ceases to amaze and delight me by the excellence of her own standards and the brilliance of her work. My gratitude, too, for the friendliness and many kindnesses of the Bear & Company staff.

I also want to pay special tribute to the Nurse Healers–Professional Associates, Inc., for permitting the use of their lists of schools where Therapeutic Touch is taught, and hospitals and health centers where it is practiced. In particular, I thank Janet Ziegler, coordinator of NH-PA, and Barbara Denison, chairperson of programs and education, who made this possible. I also appreciate the talents of Nancy Lehwalder, music therapist, who helped me understand the technical background in the harmonics of the Tibetan bells used in "Exercise of the Self 5: The Lessons of the Bells."

Finally, as always, I want to thank the generations of "Krieger's Krazies" from whom I learned abundantly, even as I taught them.

Dolores Krieger, Ph.D., R.N.
"The Rockery"
Columbia Falls, Montana
July 1996

THERAPEUTIC TOUCH
INNER WORKBOOK

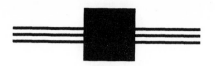

INTRODUCTION

Why Do I Want To Be Healer?

Why do I want to be healer? Why do I want to be healer? The refrain sounds in my mind with persistent rhythm. Resolutely driven, my taut limb muscles alternately shift from contraction to extension and then contract and extend again as I methodically work my way up the mountain. As though urged onward by an internal clock, in measured gait, laboriously and sometimes clumsily, my limbs seek out niche after hidden niche on that slick, precipitous incline, fingertips and toes seeking leverage in exposed tree root or embedded rock. Like a ritual dance between stolid person and questing spirit, that insistent question with its staccato cadence ratchets my body upward to the high ridge.

Perspiration of effort now and again seeps through protecting eyebrows and falls from brow into eye sockets in my upturned face so that I gauge each next step through a shimmering film of my own body fluids. I turn and am aware of you, my reader, who, like myself, may be on an interior quest. I pause, and invite you to join me in guided imagery to seek out a personal response to that unmodifiable question: *Why do I want to be healer?* I then plan to consider some major assumptions and inferences that might be drawn upon to help make personal engagement in the healing act rational, if not understandable, as a contemporary lifeway.

Guided imagery can be an excellent tool for getting to places in the psyche that often evade direct confrontation. I shall use it often in this inner workbook, which for each of us will be an opportunity to explore aspects of the inner self that engage the healing interaction.

The only prerequisite for an intriguing guided imagery experience is that you give yourself permission to interact with the up-welling imageries. My suggestion for using the guided imageries, such as the example that follows, is to either have them read to you while you close your eyes and follow the imagery, or to read them aloud into a tape recorder and then replay them as you follow the imagery. Speak clearly and at a moderately slow speed so that you will have time to follow the imagery later and respond to suggestions, and then pause a moment at the end of each paragraph for consideration of the thought. Recommendations for journaling and later analysis of your materials are found in Appendix A.

EXPLORATIONS OF THE SELF 1

Dialogue in the Cave

Materials

Pen, paper, and a tape recorder.

Procedure

Close your eyes and consider: You have become interested in Therapeutic Touch and have tried some of its techniques. You have found that you are able to help people and you wonder whether you should devote more time to its study. Should you decide to do this, you realize that you will have to refocus your worldview and perhaps change your lifestyle to accept the inevitable personal vulnerability to which compassionate concern for others will expose you. Therefore, you recognize a need to consider all aspects of why you want to become a healer before you make a final decision. In order to have the time and freedom from social constraints to examine these motivations, you decide to go off by yourself and backpack into the surrounding mountains.

You hike into the backcountry and steadily ascend the mountains. As you get to the higher elevations, the mountainsides become steeper; however, the answer to the question: *Why do I want to become healer?* still eludes you, and you persist in your ascent.

You can feel the heat of the sun on your back, and hear the clink of talus underfoot as you traverse a sharp incline. However, a glance upward assures you that you are in reach of the mountaintop and you persist, a step at a time, as your cogged movements thrust your body toward the summit.

As you top the ridge, you move a pine branch out of your line of sight and see below a long valley stretching toward the mountain that is your goal. Sweeping that mountain with your binoculars, you catch sight of a distinctive slash in the scrub growth at its base, and you use it as a guide while you descend and cross the valley.

As you near the mountain, you realize that the odd shape at the mountain's base is actually scarred terrain whose shadows indicate that it has depth. You continue closer and see that the scar apparently is the result of a recent rock slide whose slippage has uncovered a cave. You have an intimation that the cave holds a special message for you and you find yourself hurrying toward its entrance.

You go into the cave and as you do, you notice that all apprehension leaves you. You feel welcome and have a sense that you've been here before. It's cool and comfortable in the cave. As your eyes become accustomed to the subdued light beyond the mouth of the cave, you notice that it has high, vaulted walls on which are inscribed many ancient symbols, and above them are very old paintings still vibrant with brilliant coloration.

You take off your pack and, using it as a pillow, lie on the cool floor to view the paintings more comfortably. You lie back with a sigh, welcoming the slight breeze that flows from the depths of the cave. The breeze carries the gentle sound of water trickling into a pool, and for a moment you listen intently to the music of its rhythmical dripping.

You now turn all your attention to the symbols and the paintings. As you lie there, you go deeply within, center your consciousness and, staying in that quiet place, you observe them objectively and in detail.

How would you describe the mood you are in?

Is your body having any reactions to the symbols on the wall? Can you interpret your own subtle body language?

Can you sense what the pictures are saying to you? Do the pictures remind you of an experience you have had? Do the figures call to mind anyone you know?

Allow the responsive imagery to float through your mind without feeling you have to claim any of it unless a response has unmistakable meaning for you. Just relax for a few moments, look at the pictures on the wall of the cave, and let your mind work for you.

Now consider further: If you could have one question answered at this moment, what would that answer be? Take a few minutes to explore this possibility, perhaps in dialogue with anyone else you sense may be sharing this experience with you.

When you have finished your inner dialogue and while retaining what you have learned, slowly move your feet and then your hands, come back in time, and journal your impressions.

Do you now have intimations of an answer to the question: *Why do I want to be healer?* I intend to pursue the implications of this question in the following pages. Interested? Join me!

THE HUMANIZATION
OF ENERGY

A Question of Energy

"It seemed like pulsating waves of energy flowed through me. I felt strength, as though someone was standing behind and supporting me. My body felt stabilized, more in my control. I didn't think I'd ever feel like that again. It was like getting back my life."

She was describing to me how she felt when I had done Therapeutic Touch the day after she had a stroke. Since then we had set up regular sessions of Therapeutic Touch treatments. However, when we first began the treatments, eight days before, the hemiplegia that the medical doctor had diagnosed was a devastating blow to this independent woman. As she spoke my attention was riveted on the left side of her face where a week ago the facial muscles had been so flaccid that she had been unable to hold food in her mouth as she chewed and her speech was slurred. Now, her facial muscles were again symmetrical, her speech distinct, and her hemiplegia and sense of balance had cleared enough for her to get out of bed into a wheelchair with minimal assistance.

Later in the day I went down to the beach with my dogs. While I watched them play with each other as we walked the shore, my thoughts kept returning to that earlier discussion. In particular, my mind focused on the phrase, "pulsating waves of energy." I had practiced Therapeutic Touch for twenty-three years, ever since my colleague, Dora Kunz, and I first developed it. I had always thought of healing as a natural potential that anyone, with little exception, could learn to actualize. Over the years, extensive research and clinical evidence had convinced me that, in appropriate cases, Therapeutic Touch could significantly help those in need, and I had come simply to accept it as extension of my professional skills. Now, as if for the first time, I had the stunning realization that organic change had occurred during that healing process, and body tissues actually had realigned themselves and were functioning normally. Strangely, I found this to be quite an upsetting thought for, although I was involved in the healing that occurred, I realized that I didn't understand it in terms of the culture in which I lived. In this time of rationalization as an accepted way of life, I couldn't explain it.

I thought again of her words, ". . . a pulsating flow of energy." As I considered her statement, I realized that although I could accept her impression—it felt right—I really didn't know what the term "energy" meant in that context. Mulling over this thought, I whistled up the dogs and headed home. The question—*What really is energy?*—lingered in my thoughts.

EXPLORATIONS OF THE SELF 2

Energy Patterns: A Therapeutic Touch Libretto

Energy is ubiquitous. As Einstein has said, $E=mc^2$; it is everywhere and everything. It looks varied—like a fiery incandescent flash set free against the open sky, like black smoke boiling out of the confines of tall, cylindrical stacks, like a piece of iron rusting unnoticed by the wayside.

Energy is not only physical, it also runs the full spectrum of emotion, of thought, of imagination, perhaps of aspiration. It is the stuff by which we live and by which we die, the essence of all experience.

Energy is so ever-present that we become indifferent to the magic of its many guises—at the split-moment of critical mass, in a nanosecond or a wink, it can change into "the thousand and one things," and then change again and again.

In the still of these moments, we give various names to the several different kinds of energy manifestations as they are caught in the rigid mesh of time and space—an illusion, of course. To get a sense of the infinite varieties of energetic patternings, for the next few minutes just allow free rein to your imagination and be sensitive to the vivid visualizations that will arise to mind spontaneously as I recall to you a few of the ways energy patterns itself. This is done best by lightly closing your eyes, then just "go with the flow" as you hear the words in your mind, either as someone reads them to you or as you listen to the playback of a tape recording. Allow the words you hear to show you in their own way their amazingly wide range and magically diverse transformations.

Energy rays.
It streaks,
    bursts,
    thrusts.
It has projections,
    outpourings,
    pulsations.
Energy rolls in ground swells.
It has wavelets within waves,
Rippling effects spin off
    in thrills,
    shimmerings,
    iridescences.
Energy sprays, and it swirls.
Its incessant flow
    rushes,
    floods,
    ebbs.
Energy creates in myriad,
    sparkling ripples,
    rhythmic tides,
      tumbling,

twisting,

turning.

Currents of a flowing time,

set against a void

of timelessness.

Journal your impressions and any comments you have about energy, and then read on to explore further the notion of energy.

———————————————————————————————

Several days later, with my question still coming to mind whenever there was an idle moment, a few more pieces of the puzzle fell into place. I was visiting Carol and Henry, my next-door neighbors. We had shared gardening tips, handymen, and cordwood over the past three years. Now they had become pregnant and were eagerly awaiting their first child, due within three weeks. We were spending a rainy afternoon together addressing envelopes that would soon carry the announcement of the baby's birth (Martin, if it was a boy; Adriana, if it was a girl). The baby had been quite active, stretching and turning, and Carol asked me to do Therapeutic Touch to relax her, hoping that the child would also quiet down. In a short time it was a done deed, and I asked Henry if he would like to get a sense of his child's vital-energy field. Henry's eyes widened and he looked at me as though I was slightly daft.

"Come, try it," I said to him. "Do what I taught you. Just center and then assess Carol's abdomen, just as I am doing, and tell me what you are experiencing."

"Do it, Henry," Carol urged, "I want so much for you to share this experience."

That urging did, indeed, do it, and Henry slowly got up and moved toward Carol. I watched him cross the room, a quizzical expression on his face, and then stop in front of Carol. He lightly closed his eyes as he centered his consciousness and stretched his hands out toward Carol's abdomen. A moment of quiet, and then Henry's eyes opened wide in obvious astonishment.

"I felt him! I felt him!" he shouted, his voice hoarse with emotion. "I never touched him, but I felt him!" he continued.

Carol got up and hugged him, and they described their experience in bursts of half-sentences and phrases, each understood by the other.

Later, I thought of that unexpected and happy moment as I walked home. A new life was about to be born. An individual being with singularly unique traits and husky lungs would soon be proclaiming her- or himself to the neighborhood, but for now the baby still remained a silent mystery wrapped in a protective womb, another enigma. In repetition of the generations of my kind who had witnessed the blooming of pregnancy over the eons, I marveled at the true grace that attends the prenatal period.

Caught up in those thoughts of the wonderful enactment of birth, another part of my brain blinked the sober message that the one thing that would decisively mark the child's aliveness would be animation—living human energy. Intrigued by that thought, I pursued the idea. *How does the life process incorporate the kinds of energy that define life itself? How does energy enter the physical being and make it live?*

A jolt of guilt that I had probably been inattentive when this topic was covered in graduate studies carried me to my bookshelves. Texts on bioenergetics, I felt sure, would feed me the answer.

Bioenergetics, I read, is concerned with the mechanisms by which utilizable energy is generated, transferred, and manipulated to do work in biological systems. As I continued this inquiry, I realized that a major clue to the answer would be found in the unusual folding of the molecular structure of protein that enables it to function as a three-dimensional spring. Soon, a half-formed hunch was confirmed that it would be water—the wellspring of life—that would be implicated in the quickening of the protein spring.

The spring is set in motion by heat exchange as molecules of water collide with the protein and cause the protein spring to oscillate. This oscillation repetitively swings from an expanded state to a contracted state, and at the two extremes of its cycle, kinetic energy and potential energy are constantly being interconverted. At this microlevel the protein, as a unit, can be conceived as an immense storehouse of energy in three interconvertible forms: electrical, mechanical, and chemical. The theory is that as the protein molecule swings to and fro like a pendulum, the charges and dipoles are periodically separated, and, in this way, generate *electrical* energy. In the process, the relative positions of the molecules go through periodic change and thereby also generate *mechanical* energy. In addition, chemical bonds are being made and broken as the cyclic swing continues, generating *chemical* energy. Protein accounts for about 40 percent of the physical body's makeup; therefore, I could understand that these innumerable microinteractions could generate powerful internal forces in the service of the human being.

Well, OK, I thought, that's a neatly rolled-up ball of wax. Mechanistic, of course, but then there you are: You had a question, now you have an answer that can be demonstrated in a test tube. . . . Test tube? thought I. Test tube? Whatever happened to the baby?

That unexpected query prompted a tape of memories to unroll, memories of failure-to-thrive newborn babies, born prematurely and without robust vital signs, who rapidly lost all sign of crucial clinical indicators in spite of the intervention of heroic medical measures. Therefore, they had been extubated and declared dead. In several cases in the United States, nurses who were present in the neonatal intensive care units quietly picked up the apparently dead baby and did Therapeutic Touch. In too many instances to discount simply, the babies recovered and lived. As vital signs were reestablished, the children were reintubated, intravenous and other lifelines were reinserted, and the babies eventually went home to happy families.

What had happened to the protein springs in these cases where the clock had started up again? Immobile, transfixed inertia was transmuted into living, cycling ebb and flow—by what? I thought of the seemingly simple process of Therapeutic Touch that had taken place in those neonatal ICUs, and asked myself: *Where was the clue?*

Intentionality: The Necessary Mindfield Factor

Early in the development of Therapeutic Touch, Dora Kunz and I had realized that a foundational concept underlying its efficacy was that the therapist rebalanced vital energies with intentionality. The connotation of that term "intentionality" is not only that the will was involved—for example, wanting the person to get well—but there was also the implication that there is a goal in mind for the object of the intention. Logic would then suggest that Therapeutic Touch is being done as a conscious, mindful act based on a person's knowledge of the therapeutic functions of the human vital-energy field. I recaptured the visualization of engagement in the Therapeutic Touch process and recalled how, for instance, the nurses had been utilizing healing human energies to help those babies. A moment's reflection brought me to the recognition that, of course, it was the mind that had directed the flow of energy. Dynamically driven by intentionality, the clock started again, and the protein spring was again swinging through the arc of life.

EXPLORATIONS OF THE SELF 3

On Being Present: An Exercise in Intentionality

Procedure

1. Sit upright, but without strain, in a chair or on the floor, and place the palm of one hand on your lower abdomen, about three inches below the umbilicus.

2. Quietly and normally take two or three breaths nasally; meanwhile, be aware of the expansion and contraction of your abdominal muscles as you breathe:

> Inhale - pause - exhale - pause
> Inhale - pause - exhale - pause
> Inhale - pause - exhale

3. Do the exercise once more; however, this time when you exhale, bring the breath down to your lower abdomen and exhale through your hand that is placed there:

> Inhale - pause - exhale through the hand - pause
> Inhale - pause - exhale through the hand - pause
> Inhale - pause - exhale through the hand - pause

4. Journal your experience. Did you have any difficulty exhaling through your hand? What did it feel like? Can you still exhale through your lower abdomen, even though your hand is no longer there?

Comment: With minimal practice most people will have no difficulty in exhaling through their abdomen. There is no need to exert effort. We do it naturally; whenever we want to bring attention to a particular area of the body as, for instance, when we hurt, we touch it and the energy to help the hurt goes to that spot.

In the act of focusing attention with intentionality, as is done with Therapeutic Touch, we also bring energy to one area or another, as the need dictates. Therefore, to take this exercise one step further:

5. Try the last part of the exercise once more; however, this time move your hand slightly away from your body, so that there is a space between your hand and your abdomen, and be aware of what is happening in your hand chakra as you exhale.

6. Journal your experience. Could you feel the energy flow with your hand chakra? What did it feel like?

———————————————————————————————————————

This experience was not stressful. As you experienced, energy effortlessly flowed to where the mind directed. It is in this simple manner that Therapeutic Touch is directed with intentionality to an area, whether that area is part of your own body or another's. Recall again the incidents stated above about the premature babies in neonatal intensive care units. We can appreciate that the nurses doing Therapeutic Touch were not simply bereaved mother figures; their actions were guided by specific intentionality, and they tried to help intelligently. Later, we will return to this seemingly simple exercise and examine it from another point of view.

Pattern Recognition of the Vital-Energy Field

Intentionality during the act of Therapeutic Touch seems to be birthed out of the unique background effects that attend the state of continuous centering of consciousness. In some dynamic manner, perhaps best understood by masters of meditation (for which centering is a prerequisite), maintaining a centered consciousness seems to transport the mind to a deep level where patterns make sense.

Nature talks to us in patterns. In Therapeutic Touch the message is in the patterns embedded in the vital-energy field. We recognize these as cues that we term "heat", "tingling", "congestion", and "dysrhythmias", for example. It is by the subtle signals of these cues that we determine where imbalances are in the healee's vital-energy field.

Vital energies have a tendency to gather into groups or levels so that patterns result which are energetically distinct. At a physical level, these patterns are called "functional attributes." For instance, they arise in the personality as behavioral patterns whose energies translate with specificity; we call them habits, emotional dispositions, or moods. As an example, when we pick up the patterning of cues indicative of depression, they feel to our hand chakras to be heavy, unresponsive, sluggish, or congested, and without vitality. We repattern, or rebalance, these cues by relating to a principle of opposites. We would "cool" the areas where we felt heat, or "release" the pressure of congestion, or "dampen" the tingling, or "synchronize" the dysrhythmias in the healee's vital-energy field.

It is, of course, intentionality that we are using in the directing of those vital energies. The connotation here is that not only is there power as will at work, but also conscious, mindful action is innately engaged. We might even go one step further, and still be within the bounds of logic, by recognizing that the latter aspect (conscious, mindful action) presupposes a knowing relationship at some "X" level between the individual self and the object of the intended act. This makes healing a conscious, premeditated act, rather than a gut-level demonstration of impulse.

This "inner workbook" is based on the general assumption that you, the reader, are cognizant of the earlier literature on Therapeutic Touch; have put that information into practice; and, as a result, have acquired considerable personal knowledge about the Therapeutic Touch interaction. Therefore, as a useful background for the in-depth processing that will occur as you explore the following pages, I will list briefly the fundamental information most of us would agree to, based upon our experiences with, and knowledge about, Therapeutic Touch.

A Short Listing of Core Information
on the Therapeutic Touch Process

Therapeutic Touch is a contemporary interpretation of several ancient healing practices that are concerned with the knowledgeable use of the therapeutic functions of the human vital-energy field.

Within this context, Therapeutic Touch is a conscious act based upon a body of knowledge derived from logical deduction; formal and clinical research findings; a compendium of world literature concerning the therapeutic use of vital human energies; deep experiential knowledge that grows over time into a personal knowing; and tested insight.

As portrayed within the mature Therapeutic Touch process, healing is concerned with the conscious, full engagement of the therapist's own access to vital-energy flows in the compassionate interest of helping another person who is ill. Healing, then, can be thought of as a humanization of energy.

Therapeutic Touch is only concerned with vital, living energies. Primary human energies include vitality, emotion, thought, altruism, and spirituality.

Interactive vital-energy flow is a natural aspect of all living beings. It is in constant, controlled movement that is unimpeded in the healthy person.

Prerequisites of the Therapeutic Touch therapist acting as healer or human support system are that she or he have a compassionate motivation, a metaneed, to help or to heal those who are ill; the intentionality to guide the healee toward specific therapeutic goals; and the understanding of how to facilitate that healing.

The point of entry into the Therapeutic Touch process is the act of centering. The therapist remains on-center even while proceeding with other phases of the Therapeutic Touch process: the assessment, rebalancing, and reassessment of the healee's vital-energy field.

The Therapeutic Touch therapist acts as a human support system, guiding and repatterning the healee's weakened and disrupted vital-energy flow to the end that the healee's own immunological system is stimulated and recovery is strengthened and reinforced.

Working from a center of clarity is of prime importance, we can now recognize, because in responsibly intervening in another's life we must be aware of why, as well as how, we are intervening. In my own attempts to bring this steady awareness into Therapeutic Touch practice, I try to adhere to something like the following exercise, which is called the "Deep Dee". The "Deep Dee" will provide you with a simple, but elegant, device for recalling experiences that may or may not have a specific time reference, when you are engaged in the Therapeutic Touch process.

EXPLORATIONS OF THE SELF 4

Exercising the Deep Dee, Part 1

Exercise Form

PHASES OF THERAPEUTIC TOUCH:	WHAT I AM DOING:	
	Energetically:	Consciously:
Centering:		
Assessment:		
Rebalancing:		
a. Directing:		
b. Modulating:		
c. Unruffling:		
d. Other:		
Reassessment:		

Note: Your future Therapeutic Touch practice, and the welfare of your clients, will be shaped by your day-to-day Therapeutic Touch experiences. The validity of and much of the confidence in your healing ability will develop through experiential, personal knowledge. Therefore, during practice sessions it is important to look over your own shoulder, so to speak, to become consciously aware of the deep, inner processings that are playing themselves out through the Therapeutic Touch interaction.

To get a progressive sense of this personal dynamic, the "Deep Dee, Part 1" worksheet is designed to help you question yourself on at least two aspects of this self-exploration while you are doing Therapeutic Touch. Ask yourself the following questions (and put the answers into writing so that you can analyze them at a later time): What am I doing? That is, what am I experiencing energetically as I do these techniques? How am I capturing the subtle dynamics happening just beyond my skin? What sensations am I feeling, and what is my gut response to them? What is my vital-energy language saying?

Then query yourself a bit more deeply and ask: Where is my awareness focused? What is happening in my consciousness and how do I perceive it? What impressions are flowing through me? What faculties are coming into play: visualizations? fleeting ideas? appreciations? deep promptings? undoubtable insights? What are the cues that I am picking up to help me to help this person who is in need?

Comment: The trick of this exercise is to look for answers to these questions while remaining on-center. It is as if you are using both hemispheres of the brain simultaneously, finely integrating the information in real time so that you may be fully present in the compassionate interest of healing or helping.

Of course, the above-mentioned "trick" is a "coyote". These are baby steps, true. But with consistent practice, what is being exercised is an attitude of self-awareness that is oriented toward a stage of self-realization. As you get closer to your goal, another bit of the answer to "*Why do I want to be healer?*" will fall into place, and Grandfather Coyote will smile.

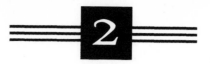

THE SET AND
THE SETTING OF
THERAPEUTIC TOUCH

Centering: Potent Ally of the Therapeutic Touch Process

Grandfather Coyote bids us, "Look! Listen!" ever deeper, bringing the fullness of mindful experience to this moment, thus letting us perceive the Therapeutic Touch process from a more fully developed perspective. In addition, as Therapeutic Touch has become more popularly accepted and variously interpreted, there has been a slight drift away from original intentions. New ideas are always worth considering; however, what has been glossed over has been the undeniable source of the empowerment of Therapeutic Touch, that decisive shift in consciousness known as "centering."

To cautiously borrow a concept from physics, unlike other healing modalities that work in series, Therapeutic Touch works in parallel. That is, Therapeutic Touch is very dissimilar to healing practices in which first one does this, and then does that, aspect of a technique. Therapeutic Touch, of course, does begin by the therapist centering his or her consciousness; the process then progresses in parallel, the centering continuing even while the Therapeutic Touch therapist is doing other things, such as assessing or rebalancing the vital-energy field of the healee. Thus, centering acts as a constant ally to all the other processes that are bound in the Therapeutic Touch interaction. Once that conscious connection is secured, there is always something or somebody—depending upon how you view your inner self—to conduct a monologue or a dialogue with in reflection, when difficult problems come up during Therapeutic Touch. As this relationship becomes an increasingly viable part of life, it can bring with it urges of creativity and promptings of intuition that we are pleased to recognize as precious facets of our real selves.

However, and unfortunately, there are many who misconstrue the reason for centering during the Therapeutic Touch process, who have been led to believe that more skills will make their practice better, sometimes the more technical, the better, they think. In reality, however, Therapeutic Touch is very much like the martial arts in that the person playing the role of healer has to be more than a master of techniques; he or she must be a master of the self. That is not only where the battle lies; it is also where the magic, the healing power of Therapeutic Touch, dwells. Techniques, in fact, are the least important part of Therapeutic Touch. In a certain sense it doesn't matter where you put your hands. What matters is how masterfully you use your mind. Thus, to be a master of yourself, it is important to know who or what it is that you master. In Therapeutic Touch it is the act of centering that undeniably holds that key; it is in quietude that we find the way to self-exploration of latent abilities, which makes Therapeutic Touch an ever-challenging, personal learning experience.

Characteristics of Centering of the Consciousness

Being on-center does not mean being still, immobile, rigid. In everyday life we are constantly reacting to other people, emotions, thoughts, and events. In centering we are quiet and "listen" to another language. Our attention goes to the heart region, where we find our own center of peace and know it as an attribute of our true self. We find that this sense of deep serenity is reminiscent of the utter peace we find in untrammeled nature and, with a thrill of personal discovery, realize that it is through such profound natural experiences that we can be at-one with the universe.

The boon of centering, however, is not only in its quieting effect. In healing it is also important to learn to put an integrated sense of being to work for us so that in the experiencing of it, we begin to understand how to offer the healee the bond of inner acceptance too. To begin such inquiry, we must be willing to acknowledge that there are several facets of consciousness, many of which lie unawakened and potential within us, awaiting an opportunity to rise to consciousness. In accepting the challenge to actualize these potentials, we actively seek out our own latent aspects. It is in this exploration of self that centering becomes the source of empowerment for the Therapeutic Touch process. How, we wonder, does this happen?

Several factors characterize this distinctive shift in consciousness. Perhaps the most prominent is a psychomotor quieting. Bodily movements become quieted almost to the point of a relaxation response. Nevertheless, we become keenly aware that an inner "listening" state is at our disposal to heed the presenting nonphysical cues of the healee's vital-energy field. This state is accompanied by a sense of timelessness. Most perceptions are usually accelerated so that we don't realize until the conclusion of the Therapeutic Touch process how little real time has passed, or some perceptions are slowed and later we are surprised to find how much time has elapsed.

Coupled with this state is a sense of inner equilibrium and well-being. Perception deepens and we are less aware, or simply not aware of the constant top-of-the-head monkey chatter of the brain. We find ready access to deep thrusts of inquiry, and this engagement of self becomes an "effortless effort" when well done; that is, it engages concentrated mind forces with no, or very little, tension involved.

Over time we recognize in ourselves a growing awareness that may blossom into intuition, and learn to have confidence in it and a respectful humility for the insistent declaration of power on its own terms. Very often a certain synchronicity enters life activities. Elevators stop and open their doors as you walk down a corridor, empty taxis pull up to the curb as you exit the building, the traffic lights get stuck in the "green-go" position as your car enters the boulevard, and in all ways your sense of timing and rhythmicity radically sharpens.

As you hone new skills and put them to work in your healing, previous allegiance to the randomness and chaos of the everyday world falters. As perspective shifts, you may begin to recognize the ordering principles underlying healing that were not apparent before. Set against this background, your worldview changes, and your out-of-step lifestyle changes in tandem. In the process, the therapist's personal ego redesigns its image, now becoming cognizant of your passion to help those in need, and of the power of compassion to move the immovable and change the immutable.

Centering as an Act of Interiority

Centering, therefore, is not a sinking into a trancelike state in which we go through motions but not know how we got there. It is, in fact, an actively conscious state. The vital-energy flow in a centered state of consciousness is the opposite of being empathic to a healee, where the healer "flows" out to the healee in an attempt to identify, and so understands this person's feelings. Centering, in contrast, is a mindful, focused act from the depth of our conscious being where the vital-energy flow gathers its forces within. Of course, at the same time, the Therapeutic Touch therapist is also empathic to the healee. Therefore, we might say that the Therapeutic Touch therapist's vital energy seemingly flows in opposite directions. However, although this would seem apparent in a 3-D logic, surely in the multidimensional domain of the nonphysical, factors such as vital-energy flow take on characteristic strangenesses that call for different nonlinear rules, and these rules can be confirmed by experience.

By remaining on-center, the healer is able to convey to the healee the sense of deep peace that presages a rapid (two-to-four minute) relaxation response as the Therapeutic Touch session proceeds. It is this profound relaxation response that facilitates the responses of the healee's immunosystem, laying an important groundwork for the

Therapeutic Touch rebalancing processes.

This act of centering, or "flip" in consciousness, permits us to be more aware of our natural selves, and to become sensitive to the natural forces around us. To get to these deep places within yourself, oddly, you need your own permission. Given permission, these facets of consciousness are there, fully present to you. In fact, from an evolutionary point of view, they want to be an active part of your life; but, psychology tells us, they need your conscious acknowledgment to be present for you. And it's worth your while to give permission, for a new awareness and a new way of life are at stake.

When you do get to that place, then you may become aware that what you are treading is, indeed, a new way, a path of self-realization of your ability to compassionately help those in need. For the Therapeutic Touch therapist that, too, is a necessary power, for it is obvious that compassion should always be a constant companion to those who would heal.

Therapeutic Touch Cues: A Language for the Future

In Therapeutic Touch, the art of "listening"—a finely focused, attentive state of becoming acutely aware of cues or hints that derive from subtle patterns in the vital-energy flows of the healee's field—is implicit in the phase of the Therapeutic Touch process known as the "assessment." Such "listening," of course, proceeds against the background of the continued centered state of consciousness previously noted. These sensed cues might be considered to be metaphors or analogies of the true state of affairs in the healee's vital-energy field. In fact, a musical analogy itself might clarify the act of "listening" through which you can pick up these cues, as in Exercise of the Self 5, "The Lesson of the Bells", below.

EXPLORATIONS OF THE SELF 5

The Lesson of the Bells

Note: What is this art of mindful "listening" that is characteristic of the Therapeutic Touch assessment? Is it possible to simulate the experience of "listening" and so practice the art? Let us try!

Materials

Pen, paper, and a set of resounding bells, such as the Tibetan bells illustrated below (figure 1).

Comment: The two sections of this bell are tuned one-half tone apart: when the two are struck against each other, one is in the tone of E and the other is E-flat. They make a clear resounding tone, the ringing sound reverberating outward in waves, each overtone awakening its unique response in the listener.

The attitude of alert, attentive listening that you assume as the resonance lowers and finally fades and you strive to hear every last

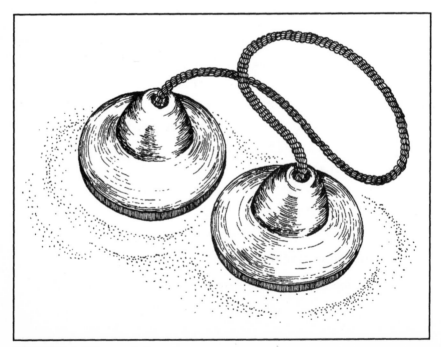

FIGURE 1: Tibetan Bells

beautiful note, is, in an analogous way, quite similar to the sensitive but vigilant state of "listening" assumed when a Therapeutic Touch therapist begins to assess subtle imbalances in the healee's vital-energy field and to map the isobars of fine variations in that ethereal territory. To fully appreciate the experience, read the brief instructions noted below, commit them to memory, and then concentrate on listening to the bells.

Procedure

1. Seat yourself comfortably, holding the bells so that they can strike each other when swung by the leather thongs.

2. Either close your eyes or, in a relaxed manner, look directly ahead with "soft" eyes.

3. Quietly center your consciousness.

4. Strike the bells together one time, and be aware of what is happening in your consciousness as you attentively listen to the bells resound. "Listen" deeply, feeling the vibrations of the sounding bells, until there is silence once again.

5. Describe what happened in your consciousness when you "listened" to the bells. Write down your impressions and, later, try this exercise with other people and discuss your experience.

Assessment of the Vital-Energy Fields

In Therapeutic Touch practice, the cues that you can become aware of with the sensitive hand chakras can take on several forms:

- breaks in energy flow
- vital-energy deficit and vital-energy hyperactivity
- a sense of pressure or fullness
- congestion or sluggishness or blockages of vital-energy flow
- dysrhythmias or random pulsations of flow
- temperature differentials of heat or cold, so innately dissimilar that variations can be clearly identified

- a sense of tinglings or slight electric shocks

- true intuitions and insights

Part of the reason for the sometimes-odd terms these cues have been given is that the English language does not have adequate descriptors for these sensed factors. This lack does seem strange, considering that ninety-three cultures in the world accept that there are essential human vital-energy fields. However, the more interesting fact is that Therapeutic Touch therapists working with this system of cues can communicate and understand each other, particularly when two or more therapists assess the same healee and then compare notes. This qualitative reliability indicates that the roots of a valid communication system describing human vital energies are taking hold. It is a communication system that crosses geographic boundaries with unexpected ease.

It has, in fact, true transcultural overtones, for at the time of this writing, Therapeutic Touch has been successfully taught in seventy-five countries.

As noted, the prime purpose of Therapeutic Touch assessment is to get a sense of the vital-energy dynamic that has gone awry in the healee's field. These are the cues the therapist's hand chakras pick up; then he or she uses this knowledge to determine how to rebalance the healee's vital-energy field. However, even as this interpretation and analysis are proceeding, the Therapeutic Touch therapist consciously and actively, but without strain or tension, seeks out the deeper levels of self in an act of interiority, as described previously.

One serendipitous result of the continued effort to help another who is ill or in need is that, as we learn to stay on-center and "listen," we also learn what makes us "tick." An "AH-HA!" or insightful experience about individual potential may then reward the therapist as these latencies are actualized over time. It is from this creative base of progressive learning about the inner self that the therapist continues to interact with the cues that arise to his or her awareness from the healee's vital-energy field, all the while trying to understand the cues, the meanings that are set against the backdrop of new personal knowledge. This field of self-interactive inquiry then becomes a "real" world of personal exploration with its own sense of timelessness and implicate order, uniquely setting the stage for individual playings out of personal growth patterns.

Therapeutic Touch cues speak a common language to those who have had such experiences. To give a sense of that experience, I have integrated a series of statements made by students during a class discussion in a course I was teaching, "Strategies of Teaching Therapeutic Touch." The statements (see below) were spontaneous; I have rearranged only the sequence of comments and added logical connections.

EXPLORATIONS OF THE SELF 6

Significant Experiential Factors that the Healer Relates To During the Assessment Phase of the Therapeutic Touch Process

Materials

Pen and paper.

Procedure

Quietly read, or have read to you, the following statements as a single, whole experience. However, pause after each paragraph and consider the statements' implications for your own practice of Therapeutic Touch. Note your reactions in your journal and discuss them when you have finished the exercise.

I am centered. I feel rooted and grounded. In the aura of protection radiating from my inner self, I am open, alert, and aware and sense the permission to allow my sensitivities their full range.

There is a sense of undisturbed weightlessness, and in this environment of profound calm, my concentration deepens. My perception sharpens and pictures float across my mind as I establish a deeper relationship with the healee.

Memories well up—AH-HA! I am aware of sensations of consciousness from the centers in the vital-energy field overlying my hands. Slight changes in the healee's personal energy, cues from energetic movement and tone, shifts in rhythm, unexpected variations of scintillating colors—all register in my mind as objective, unbiased sensory data.

I identify more closely with the healee and, lo, I'm in a timeless space! I am conscious of subtle perceptions—clear, though altered states of consciousness. The overriding compassion that I feel for the healee becomes tinged with awe and sheer joy. I feel a sense of anticipation from the healee and I am aware of the power of our rapport. This sense of oneness evokes feelings of reverence for the deep self we share—an ineffable state: words fail me.

Rebalancing the Vital-Energy Field

The way the Therapeutic Touch therapist plays out the role of healer seems to be utter simplicity itself. He or she adheres to a principle of opposites that is supported by an assumption that illness, in fact, represents an imbalance of vital energies in the sick person. This principle suggests that the charge to the therapist is to rebalance that vital-energetic state by directing or modulating vital energies qualitatively different than the cues picked up in the assessment of the healee. In various guises, this principle of opposites is universally accepted by healers around the world who work with the concept of vital energies.

For example, if the cue the therapist sensed was heat, in the rebalancing phase the sense of cool energies would be projected, and vice versa. However, the recognition of "heat" or "cold" may occur at different levels of consciousness in individual Therapeutic Touch therapists; that is, some persons may have sensed several degrees of differentiation within the categories of heat or cold, and each variation may convey subtle distinctions. The seeming simplicity of Therapeutic Touch reflects the fact that it is a human potential that can be actualized, and some people do Therapeutic Touch with ease. However, access to Therapeutic Touch does not indicate the depth at which the therapy is being done. The depth is an indication of the degree of mindfulness that illumines the therapist's expertise.

The rebalancing of any two therapists, therefore, has finely drawn differences dependent on each one's skill, knowledge, and judgment. For instance, a "hot" cue may correctly indicate to a novice that an imbalanced process was in effect. A more experienced and sensitive therapist might recognize that the cue was coupled with a background of distinctive, fine dysrhythmias. This additional information could indicate, for instance, that a disease process was ongoing. This therapist might also recognize that the tissue had been subjected to recent radiation therapy and that the cues were deeply "inth"—that is, they arose from within the intrinsic matrix of the tissues. Assessing with great care and sensitivity other areas of the healee's vital-energy field, the more experienced Therapeutic Touch therapist might critically analyze the total situation and fine-tune his or her assessment before deciding how to incorporate all of the information into the subsequent rebalancing. From time to time, and certainly before the two therapists concluded the Therapeutic Touch interaction, they might reassess the healee's vital-energy field to discern how the field was reacting to the Therapeutic Touch rebalancing. That reassessment might also give them an indication of where they should go next in the Therapeutic Touch process.

Similarly, if both of the therapists picked up a cue of "cold," they might each derive a spectrum of meaning that was also dependent upon their individual expertise. For some, "cold" might indicate a vital-energy deficit, and they would be right. However, more experienced or perceptive Therapeutic Touch therapists might also recognize other indicants, cues that might inform them more specifically. For instance, one type of "cold" might indicate that the lack of energy was caused by a dysfunctional endocrine gland, while "cold" with other qualitative differences might indicate to the therapists that some additional or deeper problem was involved in the imbalance of these fine vital energies. Much of what both therapists might do in relation to the overall cue of "cold" might be similar. However, the more knowledgeable therapist, of course, might go on to finely rebalance at levels commensurate with his or her deeper understanding. This fine-tuning ability does not contradict the notion that Therapeutic Touch therapists can communicate about these cues to each other with a great deal of clarity. It is the acuity of the communication that would differ and, just as in "real life," that difference would be relative to the situation. Each therapist would understand the other; each would perceive from the same perspective; they would share a worldview.

EXPLORATIONS OF THE SELF 7

The Worldview of Therapeutic Touch

Note: It is suggested that you use "The Worldview of Therapeutic Touch" as a guided meditation. Be sensitive to your reactions to each statement and evaluate, on the basis of your experience with Therapeutic Touch practice, whether it rings true for you.

There is an underlying integrative harmony in the universe that is reflected in the ordering principles of the healing process, and where there is order, there is meaning.

In this meaningful universe, human beings are essentially a complex of finely integrated and united vital-energy fields. In health, a fundamental law of dynamic symmetry maintains vital energies in self-regulated, balanced flow; in illness, there is a critical imbalance of those energies.

Since all living beings are open energy systems, transfer of such energies between people is a natural, passive, continuous event. When they are guided by conscious, mindful action, as in

Therapeutic Touch, specific vital energies can be projected to a healee by a healer who is moved by compassion to help or to heal another.

Therapeutic Touch is a contemporary interpretation of several ancient healing practices, and, therefore, it is transcultural in origin. It is concerned with the knowledgeable use of the therapeutic functions of the vital-energy field. Therapeutic Touch is a conscious act based on two avenues of deep inquiry. One aspect is a body of knowledge derived from logical deductions, formal and clinical research findings, a compendium of world literature concerning the therapeutic use of vital energies, and an experiential knowing that grows over time into a personal knowledge. Conjunctive to the latter and often developing concomitantly with it, the consistent practice of Therapeutic Touch becomes an interior experience for the therapist by way of an exploration of the deeper reaches of self during the act of centering the consciousness. Although the basic techniques of Therapeutic Touch are both natural and simple, its more advanced techniques are dependent upon the willingness and ability to study in considerable depth your own being during the healing act. It is then that the internal dynamics of this act of interiority impel an upwelling of compassionate response that clearly sounds the imperatives of the higher orders of self. This upwelling reflects within you a rising sense of empowerment to help or to heal self and others, and an increasing confidence in that healing enactment.

Therapeutic Touch therapists use touch as a telereceptor; that is, the therapist most frequently works at a distance from the body, in the healee's vital-energy field, rather than by directly contacting the skin's surface. In this way, the healer telereceives information about the healee's condition—the healer's perceptual ability acts over a distance in response to subtle vital-energy cues in the healee's field. These cues appear to be the result of changes in the vital-energy patterns. The Therapeutic Touch therapist does not "go out" to the healee, for instance, as in empathic response, but rather goes "inth," deeply within, in an act of interiority that probes the higher orders of self for insights into healing ways to meet the needs of the healee.

Acting as a compassionate support system, the healer guides and repatterns the healee's weakened and disrupted vital-energy flows so that his or her own immunological system will be stimulated, recuperative abilities will be restored, and vital energies will once more be in harmonic balance. It is the healee who fundamentally heals him- or herself, for human beings have as much natural potential to transform their own personalities and to transcend their personal life conditions as they do to compassionately help or heal one another.

Theoretical Background of Contemporary Healing

Every worldview rests on the philosophy of its time. Briefly, in the mid-1970s, major insights into the validity of healing set the background for a surging interest in the nature of human potential for person-to-person helping and healing. The groundwork was laid by extensive studies by Krippner on transcultural bases for para-nor-mal activities (1980), and on shamanism and healing (Krippner and Vollodo, 1976). Within a short span of time these and derivative works stimulated intensive explorations on the nature of self-healing (Simonton, Simonton, and Creighton, 1978); Pelletier, 1977). LeShan's work on healing at a distance and on the effects of prayer was seminal (1974). Simultaneously, the Greens began their study of internal states of biofeedback on the autonomic nervous system (1977); Tart brought to notice the range of specific states of consciousness (1975); Krieger demonstrated the effects of Therapeutic Touch on human physiological indices (1975) and introduced the notion of consciously exercising the higher orders of self as an extension of professional skills in the health sciences (1979); and Kunz described how the dynamism of the inner self reacted to illness and healing.

Much of the rationale for these studies was undergirded by Capra comparing findings of the new physics with ancient teachings on the metaphysics of the universe (1975). This work was bolstered by Pribram's recognition of the similarity of brain storage mechanisms and holographic theory (1976); that theory was further developed by Bohm's insight into a holographic universe made up of both implicate and explicate orderings (1980). Later, Sheldrake bridged the gap between the new physics and humans by conceptualizing the use of morphogenic fields that are neither space- nor time-bound for human perception and functioning.

Work on the effect of stress and mood on neuropeptides throughout the body clarified the critical interrelationships between the neurophysiology of the body and its psychological states, and immunological defense system. This recognition of endorphins and enkephalins outside the brain supported the work of the Simontons and Creighton (1978), and also Achterberg and Lawlis (1978), that had demonstrated the ameliorative effects of creative imagery on persons with malignancies. These insights were foundational in the development of a psycho-neuro-immunological view of the healing that pervades the field today (Ader, 1986).

Integrating the major findings of these seminal studies, the following is a brief statement of the theoretical foundation that underlies healing in our time.

There is significant consonance between ancient sages' perceptions of the universe and its functionings and that of the new physics. Physically, human beings are logically organized into systems and subsystems or, as seen from the personal view, these levels of organization are human vital-energy fields that are finely coordinated localizations within appropriate universal fields. A unified transcultural conception of a psychic continuum, or psychodynamic field between people, can be stated, and this continuum can be used to heal others during ecstatic trance and at a distance.

Human vital-energy fields under conditions of heavy and continued stress may lose the finely tuned rhythmicity of their integral relationships, and this dyssynchronous state allows the human vital-energy field to be vulnerable to sickness and disease. Healing per se arises out of the depths of the unconscious, and the effects of healing have physiological and psychological correlates. Remote autonomic nervous system functions can be consciously controlled. Neuropeptides that regulate pain and mood are distributed throughout the body and respond to vivid imaginative perceptions. These perceptions can be used to dissociate from pain and to stimulate the healing process.

The deep structures of the brain are thought to be analogous to a hologram. Each facet of the brain participates in the whole, and is sensitized by the universal principles of its implicate, or enfolded order of "what is to be," and its explicate, or unfolded referents to "what is." This statement of coherent ordering is a detailed reflection of ancient teachings. One of these aspects, essentially creative in nature, acts as a biofield phenomenon for communications over distance between human beings. The human being is a localized, dynamic intersection of several principal field forces that span a spectrum of vitality, life force, and creative living energies. At the core is the inner self of the individual being. From this central, ever-pulsating, vital radiation, the unique warp and woof of each lifetime is spun. It is the same loom that will provide the answer to: *Why do I want to be healer?*

3

CENTERS OF
HUMAN CONSCIOUSNESS

The Chakras As Teacher

"What does love feel like?" I find myself asking. It is easy to define: an interior feeling of deep affection or fondness for a person or thing. "A great liking," says the dictionary, "to delight in, admire, greatly cherish." Yes, of course . . . but what does love feel like? It is a tender feeling, an adoration, an intense emotional relationship. It is "an instant thirst of enjoying a greedily desired object," in the words of Montaigne; "a spiritual coupling of souls," says Ben Jonson; "what makes the world go 'round with that worried expression," quipped the ageless comedian, Fred Allen.

As far back as history records, love was regarded as a goddess. Love was a sexual love, defined in terms of fertility and worshipped for its ability to assure the grandchildren and the perpetuation of the people. Astarte of the Phoenicians identified with Isis of the Egyptians and became Aphrodite, who was born out of the foam of the sea and transformed into Venus, she who could be seen in the sky as morning star and, later, as evening star. It was all in the perspective one had, it would seem. But, in fact, neither definition nor myth answers the question: "What does love feel like?"

Why these mind wanderings? I had been studying about the human chakra's nonphysical human energy structures in the vital-energy field and the psychodynamic field of the personal self that are sources of different kinds of consciousness, and wondering how to apply what I was learning to healing. I did not "see" these subtle energies of the personal self, although my colleague, Dora Kunz, did. She was born with that ability, the fifth generation in her family to have such perception. Since a child, she has developed her abilities in self-disciplined studies, and has used these finely honed perceptual skills in her work with scientists, medical specialists, psychologists, and professional nurses, myself among them, in our development of Therapeutic Touch. Her work is of a highly skilled and unique nature (Kunz, 1985; Karagulla and Kunz, 1989; Kunz, 1991). However, as noted, I do not have these abilities, and so have had to rely on experiential knowledge, meditation, and analytical devices to capture some understanding of the dynamics of human-energy fields. Then, to satisfy myself that these notions had validity and after assuring the safety of the healee, I tested out these ideas as I was doing Therapeutic Touch.

While I was doing this testing I engaged in the colloquy on love noted above, for, at that time, I was studying the heart chakra. Although I had found that—just as in books on neurology—many books on the dynamics of the chakras read as though they were copied word-for-word from those that had been published previously, I had decided to go with a point of agreement that I had noted among them: One of the qualities characteristic of the heart chakra was love. I had rationalized that if I could understand these qualitative aspects, I would have a clue to their source.

Finally I decided to do the obvious. I quietly centered my consciousness, thought of someone I truly loved, and tried to become acutely aware of the effect that the love I was trying to express had on the various facets of my being. It was out of such quests, incidently, that the "Deep Dee" exercises (pp. 18-19, 148-152) developed. In this instance, when I thought of someone I truly loved, I found that there was a softening of my affect and a slight smile played about my lips. My energies were quietly outgoing and directed toward the object of my love. It was a pleasurable feeling, and I wanted to share myself and all I had with my loved one and be in that person's presence. My love was so overwhelming that I knew that nothing could come between me and my beloved; my love was an irresistible force. In time I realized that love, and, in fact, all emotions, were potent energies whose forces could be directed and modulated to fit the occasion. Under mindful guidance, they could become powerful allies in both self-healing and the healing of others.

Later, I conducted a three-year study (1989-1991) on the patterns of thought and symbolic images that people use to protect themselves—that is to say, their vital-energy fields—during close interactions with others (such as what occurs during the healing act). I found that the most potent way for the healer to break through these shielding barriers was by the projection of love (Krieger, 1993). Becoming aware of a flow of love from the healer, the healees, often to their surprise, found themselves eagerly accepting the proferred help and opening to the healing process.

In my search to understand the heart chakra, I used all the information I received experientially and from my studies; and, as noted above, I began to practice the intentional projection of those qualities of energy flow that I understood represented love. I would use these growing abilities while doing Therapeutic Touch, and include in my notes on each session both my subjective and objective observations on the effects of the projection of love. Coupled with meditations on love as a process, this period of intensive study added considerably to my understanding of how to help people to heal, particularly those who were in fear or panic. In addition, I found it beneficial to use these energies when working with healees who were wary or apprehensive, or who—in a few cases—were initially openly hostile to me. I also found these methods of projection helpful when supporting the healee's immunological system. In this instance, I worked with the vital-energy field overlying the thymus of those with cancer or AIDS, previous to and during chemotherapy and bone marrow transplants. Work with the heart chakra has been especially valuable in helping those who were dying through their final transition.

In working through these Therapeutic Touch procedures, I began to recognize that I was engaged in at least a two-step process. One facet had to do with the energy flows of love as feeling; however, underlying that there was a specific state of consciousness of which these feeling states were but an attribute. I now tried to align myself with that consciousness as well as with the energy flow. It was during this latter stage of my self-study that I realized that I could not study a chakra in isolation. The chakras act as sensitively coordinated networks of different kinds of consciousnesses. At their core, the chakras are integrated and intimately related to one another; therefore, the network acts in a united and coherent fashion that defies partial manipulation.

A Study of Compassion

This understanding was a significant insight for me, and compassion became the quality that I chose for further study. Conceptually, compassion encompasses both love, an aspect of the heart chakra, and aspiration, an aspect of the throat chakra. So compassion seemed well suited for the study, even from afar, of how chakras work in relation to one another. As has been the case since my earliest interest in healing, I felt my way by taking a sporting chance on decisions or ideas that seemed to well up from deep within and, in a sense, I bet my life on them. I would put these decisions or ideas to work in my life and then maintain awareness of how they affected events. I took particular note of how the conscious development of compassion for those who were in distress acted upon the happenings in my life, as well as my attitudes and moods and, of course, on the effect my Therapeutic Touch practice had on the healees with whom I worked.

My final conclusions were difficult to parse out; however, I did become convinced that the two-step process previously noted was, in fact, going on at a subtle, but cognizable, level. One level of consciousness could quite easily determine energy flows, note their characteristics in reference to illness or well-being, and have a fairly intelligent understanding of their dynamics as a process. However, underlying this level there was going on a whole other complex level of organization of which the energy flows were but a substratum. This latter aspect played itself out more and more frequently in the Therapeutic Touch process, as wellings up of insights about the healee's condition; as intuitive, correct knowings about the origins of the conditions; or as the predisposing factors that led up to their manifestation in the healee's lives. That, I later realized, was a completely different cognitive level of operations, one I had only occasionally glimpsed previously. As I learned to handle these deeper personal knowledges, I gained considerable confidence with my Therapeutic Touch practice. This, in turn, served to strengthen the understanding of my relationships with the healees with whom I worked.

I studied this unfolding of consciousness as objectively as I could during the Therapeutic Touch sessions, and for several years did not say anything to anyone about it; however, I did keep notes as I added other chakras to my self-study, and I did continue to meditate on my findings. This latter practice was especially helpful, because during meditation I felt free to search out deep places within myself, and this self-search seemed to tap wellsprings of a different perspective on the healing process. To assure that I maintained the objectivity I felt was necessary, I sought out challenging situations that would confront these insights about the healee's condition. Over time, it became a habit to request that information on the healee be kept from me so that I would be forced to make the "Deep Dee" assessment of the healee's condition unaided. I held to this convention whenever and wherever I was asked to demonstrate Therapeutic Touch. The challenges served to muster my best efforts to the moment, and I learned a lot, quickly, in the process.

EXPLORATIONS OF THE SELF 8

The Warrior of Healing, an Exercise in Compassion

Materials

Paper, pen, and the "Deep Dee" exercise form (see p. 18).

Procedure

1. Sit comfortably, and center your consciousness.

2. When you feel centered, quietly go back in your mind's eye to someone who truly loved you in such a deep manner that it moved you and caused an emotional reaction, possibly a reciprocation within you.

3. Feel that moment once again, allowing it to strongly stir your emotions, even if that person is no longer alive.

4. Clearly visualize that person as though you were standing next to him or her. Feel this person's presence as you once knew it, and reexperience the feeling of the love that once bound you to each other.

5. Turn your attention now to your respirations, and, for a moment, simply note the rhythmic motions of your breathing, as you return to the present time.

6. Now, on your next exhalation, focus on the region of your heart chakra and allow it to be open and aware. As you feel its sensitivity respond, quietly direct the energies you know as love to flow to someone you now love. Spend a moment in that outward flow of love.

7. On the next exhalation, broaden that flow of love to include all people you know. Gently keep that love flowing for the next two or three exhalations.

8. Now, extend that feeling of love to all people in need of love—the unloved, the unwanted, the forsaken, the rejected.

9. Speak to them in your mind and let them know they are not forgotten, that you recognize your link to them as another being,

and that you give this love freely, without conditions or attachments.

10. Now, think of some figure who represents that kind of love—The Mother of the World, Quan Yin, Mary, Mother Teresa, your mother, your Teacher, your Guide—and know that you are a Warrior on their Path.

11. Visualize yourself being part of their flow of compassion to the unloved and the forgotten on this planet.

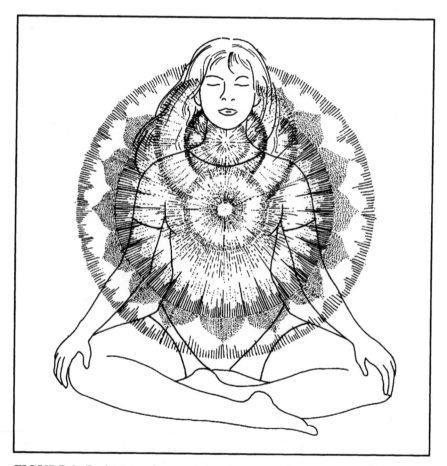

FIGURE 2: Radiation of compassionate energy from the heart and throat chakras

12. Gently and effortlessly keep that compassion flowing, and then come back when you feel ready.

13. After a moment or two, note your observations on your "Deep Dee" form, and then translate your impressions more fully into your journal.

Although until this day I do not "see" either the human energy fields of the personal self or the chakras embedded within them, I believe the events noted above have been an extremely useful exercise in my becoming aware of how these fields of consciousness play through me, and how I can continue to develop my sensitivity to them so that I can access valuable insights into the helping of others. However, please note—this learning process does acutely sensitize you to the emotions of others as well as to yourself. Therefore, although I do recommend pursuing this track of inquiry, I also caution that simultaneously you must be willing to strive toward inner balance and equilibrium in your own life. Otherwise the focused strength gained from exercising this inner exploration can constellate these forces against the person who permits the entrance into his or her life of uncontrolled emotional storms that distort and wreak havoc on the necessary calm and equanimity that attends inner listening. My sense is that my own self-study of these fields of consciousness is only in its beginning stages. Now and again through experiential, personal knowledge, I seem to catch a glimpse of their unimaginable workings; however, I know I have not yet gained a true understanding of their singular definition.

To gain a personal, but objective, appreciation of an energy-field experience, the "magneT-Touch" game was devised to challenge you in the Explorations of the Self 9. While playing this game, think of the universal magnetic field as being analogous to the universal field of human consciousness that lights up the actions of all people. The individual magnet you are stalking is a localization of the universal magnetic field and analogous to the localized field of human consciousness, the chakra complex of the individual.

EXPLORATIONS OF THE SELF 9

Fielding the magneT-Touch

A. How to make a magneT-Touch bracelet

Materials

2 small magnets, approximately 1 square inch each; cotton cloth, approximately 2-1/2 square inches; elastic material, approximately 1/2 inch by 4 inches; needle and thread.

Procedure

1. Lay out the piece of cloth and place one magnet at its center.

2. Fold side A over magnet 1.

3. Fold side B so that magnet 1 is snug against the previous fold.

4. Sew around magnet 1 with a simple overhand stitch to keep it from moving.

5. Take the length of elastic material, insert one edge into the fold at C, and sew it firmly into place.

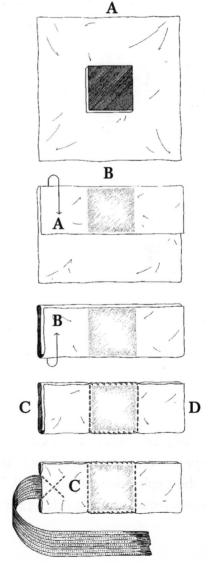

FIGURE 3: Magnet series, steps 1-5
(step 6 on p. 46)

6. Take the remaining end of the elastic material, insert it into the edge of the fold at D, and sew it into place so that you now have a magneT-Touch bracelet.

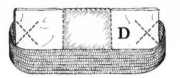

7. The magneT-Touch bracelet is worn on the hand so that the magnet is in the middle of the player's palm, at the site of the hand chakra.

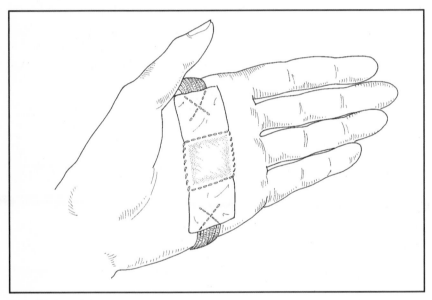

FIGURE 4: Magnet series, step 7

B. How to play magneT-Touch

Note: This is a competitive game, as well as a technique to help you get a sense of the real but invisible forces of the magnetic field.

The game can be played by either two people or two teams of equal numbers. With practice, the technique can be honed to a fine art, at which time the playing field should be lengthened or blindfolds should be placed over the players' eyes to provide further challenge. Expertise is gained by trying to sensitize your hand chakra's response to the magnetic field.

Materials

2 magneT-Touch bracelets; 2 magnets, each approximately 1 inch square. These will be called magnet 2; one will be used by each player or team.

Flat, smooth playing surface, such as a bare table. The playing field should be marked to end about one foot in front of the player. A starting mark can be placed near the edge where the players will be.

Scorecard marked:

PLAYER/TEAM: MOVES: GOALS:

Procedure

1. Each player, or team, lines up near the playing field. The players alternate in playing magneT-Touch, the beginning player/team decided by a toss of a coin.

2. To play the game, the player puts on the magneT-Touch bracelet, and approaches the playing field, on the edge of which he or she places magnet 2. The upper side of magnet 2 should be of the pole opposite that of the magneT-Touch bracelet, so that they will attract one another when placed in close proximity.

3. Placing the hand wearing the magneT-Touch bracelet near magnet 2, the player tries to move magnet 2 toward and across the finish line, one foot away. Each time the magnet is moved in any direction, it is noted on the scorecard, Each time magnet 2 is maneuvered over the finish line, a goal is scored.

4. Should the player get too close to magnet 2 so that it is captured by the magneT-Touch bracelet, the player loses his or her chance to the other player or team. Each player gets a chance to play a total of three times.

5. The object of the game is to score the most amount of goals with the least amount of moves. However, special notice is given that, in the event that a player is able to balance magnet 2 perfectly midway between the drag of the gravitational field and the attraction of the magnetic field so that magnet 2 levitates, that person

is declared a Grand Master of magneT-Touch and automatically wins the game!

———————————————————

Well, so much for fun and games. Now I would like to turn your attention to a serious consideration of the crucial part chakras, the centers or power sources of consciousness in a human being, play in the mature, conscious practice of Therapeutic Touch. The process, I am sure, will clarify your motivation to answer: *Why do I want to be healer?*

THE REALITY
OF THE CHAKRAS

Barring experiential and personal knowledge, then, how do we objectively know how the energies "out there" in the universe become a human being? The West has had little to tell us of this common, but wondrous, phenomenon. However, finally the day has arrived when, through findings in widely diverse fields—such as quantum physics and deep-space astronomy, anthropology, and animal communication—it has been generally accepted that electrons, the ancients, and perhaps space people, but certainly dolphins, whales, wolves, grizzly bears, and gorillas have unique methods of communication that, in their own realms, are quite as valid as those of human beings. Although such fields come from different perspectives, all have agreed to recognize that there is not only one reality, but several realities on this planet, an amalgam that is operating in the same space and time, but perhaps in optional conceptual frames or dimensions.

The nonordinary reality that both healers and mystics have claimed as their field of operation, however, has been long recognized and has formed a body of literature for at least the past 3000 years. Specifically, it includes the Rg Vedas (*veda* means "wisdom" or "science" in Sanskrit), the oldest literature of the East Indian people. The Rg Vedas contain the Upanishads, within which are definitive descriptions of the nonphysical chakras in the human being. Subjective descriptions of the inner dynamics of the chakra complex are impressively detailed and include how chakras act to synchronize, direct, and distribute vital energies from the various supraphysical fields in which they have had their birth to the organs of the physical body where, through their functionings, they produce various states of consciousness.

It should be noted that, although the findings about chakras are most explicitly stated in the Upanishads, descriptions of their attributes are found in the teachings of other cultures as widely geographically separate as the Sufis of the Middle East and the Native Americans, particularly in the North American Southwest. Interestingly, Western culture has inadvertently carried information through time on the chakras in the form of the well-publicized logo of the medical profession, the caduceus. On this ancient symbol, the points of contact of the two entwining snakes around the rod, which symbolizes the spinal column, represent the loci of the five major nonphysical chakras that are related to the trunk of the human body, in field contact at the vital-energy level, with a nonphysical aspect of the spinal cord called *sushumna* (Skt.). The two wings above the snakes' heads represent the two nonphysical petals or energy spirals of a sixth chakra, which overlies the pituitary gland in the brain.

To present authoritative information about the chakras, I will restrict myself to two sources. Avalon (1916), an English scholar, was the first to translate, from Sanskrit into English, ancient manuscripts that describe laya-yogic investigations of the major chakras. His works, which have been world acclaimed and won him a knighthood (as Sir John Woodroffe), will be my source of information on the traditional literature. I will add material I have learned from Dora Kunz, or which is found in her numerous writings. She is an acknowledged contemporary authority on the clinical aspects of chakra dynamics. At the end of this chapter, I will add a few general comments out of my experience with Therapeutic Touch.

Chakras as Centers of Consciousness

The chakras are centers of consciousness (*caitanya*, Skt.), writes Avalon (p.115). The sense in which their dynamic functions are described is analogous to that of localized energy fields, whose functions reflect the universal fields from which they derive. The attributes of the chakras at the level of the individual then can be expressed as foci for different kinds of consciousness that are embedded in the human energy fields of the personal self. The human energy field per se is a complex of many interpenetrating energy fields (including the electromagnetic field, the gravitational field, and the weak and strong nuclear forces), whose characteristic properties interrelate and form a unitive, living pattern, the expression of which we know as human nature. The chakras act as transformers, converting subtle-energy systems (for example, *pranas*, Skt.) into the kind of energies that make the psychophysiological being of the personal self what it is.

There are three principal forces that flow through the chakras: vitality, life force, and a potentially creative force called *kundalini*. There are several prime and secondary chakras; however, we will be more specifically concerned with the seven major sites at the level of the vital-energy field, the level that patterns the physical body in states of wellness and illness. These major chakras relate to sites at the crown of the head (the *sahasrara*, or crown chakra); overlying the pituitary gland within the brain (the *ajna*, or brow chakra); within the medulla oblongata at the conjunction of the brain and the spinal cord (the *visshuddha*, or throat chakra); and lower in the trunk of the body at the regions of the heart (the *anhata*, or heart chakra); the solar plexus (the *manipura*, or solar plexus chakra); the spleen (the spleen chakra); and at the base of the spine (the *muladhara*, or root chakra). Two of these, the crown chakra and the spleen chakra, are said not to be chakras in the usual sense of that term, and these differences will be discussed below.

Of these seven chakras, as noted, five relate to the trunk of the physical body. The sixth, the ajna chakra (*ajna*, Skt.: order or command), relates more fully to a region between the eyes, in the cavernousa nerve plexus. The sahasrara or crown chakra is frequently represented by a thousand-petaled lotus (*sarasrara*: thousand). In one of its several functions, it works together with the brow chakra in their relation to the pituitary-pineal axis. It also corresponds to the cerebrum of the brain, and is concerned with all realms of consciousness.

It is said that, ascending from the base of the spine to the top of the head, there is an increasing differentiation in both the vibratory role and in the functioning of the chakras. This results in more subtle awarenesses being brought into consciousness as a person gains successive control of the higher chakras, progressing cephalically from the heart chakra to the crown chakra.

At the base of the genitals, above the muladhara or root chakra, is the site that is somewhat outside the present discussion, the *svadhisthana* chakra. Its functions are concerned with the body's organs of secretion and reproduction. Although some regard its reproductive functions and its control of the genitourinary system to be combined with that of the next highest chakra, the manipura, if, for the sake of simple illustration, the svadhisthana is included with four of the chakras related to the trunk of the physical body, these five will each be seen to correspond to specific plexes in the surrounding nerve tissues at the sites where they impinge on the spinal cord (Avalon, p. 153), as figure 5 makes clear.

In figure 5, the muladhara (root) chakra relates to the vital-energy field overlying the sacral nerve plexus, and is in the coccygeal region; the svadhisthana chakra relates to the prostatic plexus in males and is in the sacrum; the manipura (solar plexus) chakra corresponds to the epigastric plexus and is in the lumbar region; the anahata (heart) chakra is concerned with the cardiac plexus and is in the dorsal region of the spinal cord; and the visshuddha chakra relates to the pharyngeal plexus and is in the cervical area of the spinal cord.

These chakras relate to both the central nervous system and the cranial nerves, and they affect the subtle energies of the secretory, sensory, and motor centers. They correlate to physical functions through intermediate conductors in the following way:

Chakra:	Related Physiological Function:
muladhara (root)	generation
svadhisthana	micturation
manipura (solar plexus)	digestion
anahata (heart)	cardiac action
visshuddha (throat)	respiration
ajna (brow)	visualization
sahasrara (crown)	volition

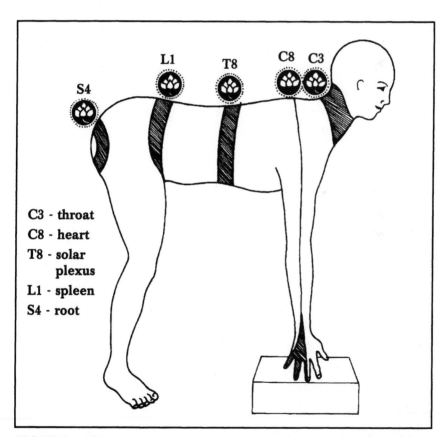

FIGURE 5. The relation of five chakras to specific nerve dermatomes of the physical body

Nadis as Human Energyways

The vitality, or vital force (prana) for these actions is carried by nonphysical structures called petals, radiating from the chakras. They are concerned with the formation and distribution of nonphysical conduits, the *nadis* (Skt. *nad*: motion), at the center of the chakra (Avalon, p. 95). The major nadi is called the *sushumna*, which goes up the spinal cord. It is said that there are two finer levels or dimensions of organization within sushumna: the first finer level is called *Vajrini*, and within the Vajrini is the *Chitrini*, which is ". . . as fine as a spider's thread." It is upon Chitrini that the chakras are threaded ". . . like gems." Sushumna rises up the spinal cord and passes into the ventricles of the brain (p. 149), extending, therefore, from the root chakra at the base of the spinal cord to the crown chakra at the top of the head. Accompanying sushumna are the two next major nadis, called *ida* and *pingala*. They relate to the sympathetic nervous system chains of ganglia running down each side of the spinal cord (p. 107). One of their important functions is to regulate breathing.

Major Chakras in the Vital-Energy Field

Using the physical body as reference, at the bottom of the spinal cord, in the root chakra, rests the latent creative force, kundalini, who ". . . maintains all breathing creatures" (p. 118). In fact, all of the nadis, 72,000 in number, arise from this site in the root chakra, which, as a complex, is called the *kanda* (p. 164). The location of the root chakra is said to be midway between the anus and the genitals for males, somewhat different for females.

Briefly, the solar plexus chakra relates to the umbilicus and, in fact, a variant of its name in Sanskrit is the *nabhisthana* chakra (*nabhi*, umbilicus). It is accorded roles in the menstrual flow, the sense of sight, the breath, and the transmission of organic substances into the psychic energies of the more sensuous emotions.

The spleen chakra is concerned with the specialization, subdivision, and distribution of prana (vitality) that comes from the sun. The functioning of the spleen chakra, however, is disturbed by fatigue, sickness, and extreme old age. Prana per se has five subsystems that can be assimilated by our bodies at this present stage of evolution. Avalon says, "It is the collective Prana that holds it (the physical body) together as a human unit, just as it supports the different principles and elements of which it is composed" (p. 161).

The heart chakra is the seat of prana, the life energy, and of the *jivatman*, the individual soul. It is ". . . the place where sages hear the pulse of life." *Vayu*, the major element to which prana is related, has its center in the heart chakra. Activation of this chakra is said to stimulate the sensitivity of touch (p. 120).

The throat chakra is the seat of *udana*, one of the five pranic subsystems mentioned above (see figure 6, page 78). It is associated with the breath that ". . . carries the soul to the head" during the state of *samadhi*, or deep, mystical "at-onement" with the source of life. It is also the site of transformation of prana through mantric power, which is the power of controlled sound. Besides sound, or because of it, the throat chakra is importantly related to both vibration and the skin.

As previously noted, the brow chakra works together with the most subtle center of consciousness, the crown chakra. It refers to the pituitary-pineal axis, and is related to the cavernousa nerve plexus. It is the seat of cognitive senses that lead to insight, clear visualization, and the more subtle senses of perception. The three major nadis mentioned above—the sushumna, ida, and pingala— braid together at the brow chakra to form a "knot," or *granthis* (Skt.). This is one of three highly important sites in the body. The other two "knots," sites of tremendous vital force, are at the heart chakra and the root chakra (p. 126).

The crown chakra also relates to the cerebral cortex, the seat of voluntary action, acts of will and altruism, and states of unitary consciousness (p. 149). The crown chakra is the goal toward which kundalini directs itself when it is activated from its usual state of latency.

Ultimately all chakras are related directly to the higher orders of the self, the inner self. These fields of consciousness have various attributes of human behaviors and, as is the case in all religious systems, the yogin treads the path of attainment by bringing these behaviors under control for some altruistic purpose. During the process of this undertaking, the nadis come into play with the goal of activating kundalini. As this is accomplished (no easy task!), kundalini begins to ascend the major nadi, sushumna. Where it accesses the three knots or granthis at the root chakra, the heart chakra, and the brow chakra, specific changes occur in the consciousnes of the seeker.

The Chakras and Their Role in Health and Illness

I drew my materials for this section from notes taken while learning directly from Dora Kunz over the past twenty-three years about the subtle effects of the chakras on the healing process, or from reading her books (Kunz, 1985; Karagulla and Kunz, 1989; Kunz, 1991). The remarks that follow appear only with her permission. Dora Kunz has a vast storehouse of personal experiences and a deep knowledge of the supraphysical worlds about which she teaches with uncommon wisdom and in an unimitable style. It is suggested that you consult her books directly for a fuller picture of the intricate dynamics of the supraphysical.

The human energy fields, Dora Kunz notes, are local representations of universal life fields. The energy flows of the vital-energy field circulate in close proximity to the physical body. There also is a psychodynamic field within the domain of the personal self which is characterized by the full range of human emotions, and a conceptual field, out of which arises abstract thought, theory, concepts, and ideas. We are individually linked to fields of other energies, such as the intuitional from which we draw our insights, and fields related to our spiritual nature. All interpenetrate one another, but each functions in its own space. Although their movements and functions are finely integrated, each field has its own specific qualities.

The chakras are found within these fields. They act as transducers, regulating the frequencies and rhythms of the field energies that flow through their core structures, while also linking the individual energy flows between the various levels of these human energy fields.

From the perspective of the individual, personal self, the vital-energy field, the psychodynamic field, and the conceptual field are of tangible and immediate importance. The vital-energy field is in continual interaction with the person's physical body, which, itself, is an intricately organized set of constantly interacting and interdependent physical energy systems. The whole complex is exquisitely integrated and serves to impregnate the physical body with life force through its lifetime relationship with its localized vital-energy field. The vital-energy field is therefore the interactive medium for the body's access to prana, which actually activates and vitalizes it.

The psychodynamic energy field is next highest in frequency, and is characterized by emotions, moods, impressions, feelings, and sensations that importantly affect the flow of energies to the vital-energy field and, through it, the physical body. At a still-finer level of organization is the conceptual field, which also can have a direct effect on the physical body, if it is not waylaid or blocked at the psychodynamic level by tangled emotions.

In a rhythmic processing that Kunz states is analogous to respiration, the vital energy from the chakras in these localized fields enters the physical body through supraphysical extensions to the spinal cord, and so is connected to the body's nervous system. These intermediary extensions connect with sushumna, the major nadi, through which prana flows. Eventually these energies return to the chakra complex and spiral out to the chakra's periphery, there to gradually meld into the supraphysical vital-energy field. In this way the subtle energies once again become part of the universal field in a constant rhythmic intake, processing, and outflow that serves to engage and organize the human energy fields of the personal self (Karagulla and Kunz, 1989; p. 36).

Thus, the life process is an intricate and complex network of vital energies and levels of consciousness. The physical body is elegantly responsive to this process, being shaped, coordinated, and vivified by the integrated actions of these energies. Disturbances or obstructions that drastically alter the normal patterns of energy flow result in loss of vitality and in ill health (p. 36).

The Supraphysical Level

The Crown Chakra

The chakras are of major importance at the supraphysical level, where they act as the principal agents for focusing energy to the physical body (p. 33). At that level the prime attribute of the crown chakra which, as noted, is directly allied with the inner self, is that of synthesizer; it relates to all of the chakras and works with all of them, most particularly those under stress or imbalance. It is, therefore, useful to bring the functions of the crown chakra into appropriate Therapeutic Touch practices, because it casts a spiritual quality over all it interacts with, particularly in times of crisis.

To understand how to work at the supraphysical level during Therapeutic Touch, try to connect with your own inner self, and talk mind-to-mind to the healee in an attempt to strengthen him or her. Although specific methods are still in the developmental stage, it may be useful to try Therapeutic Touch in this way with persons who have Alzheimer's disease, and to possibly break through to those who are mentally retarded, have epilepsy, or are autistic.

This process is also most helpful in supporting those who are dying through a peaceful final transition.

The Brow Chakra

The brow chakra functions together with the crown chakra in a unique manner, and, therefore, it is often regarded as part of it. The brow chakra has two parts, or "petals," whose functions are somewhat analogous to the neurophysiology of the two parts of the pituitary gland, with which the chakra is linked. The brow chakra is particularly concerned with the integration of ideas, the ability to visualize, and the capacity for organization. Because of the last function, it may be useful to gently, and for short periods of time, focus Therapeutic Touch practices in the brow area when working with persons with dyskinesia. In an attempt to help strengthen visualization and clarify ideas, it might be useful to consider the brow chakra in Therapeutic Touch practices with elderly persons, as well as to foster the integration of ideas for those with attention deficit. Additionally, there are the neurophysiological functions of the organs, such as the pituitary, to be considered. Therefore, it is appropriate to study Therapeutic Touch practices to alleviate the effects of bone malformations, or poor absorption of calcium, such as occur in osteoporosis. As in all Therapeutic Touch practices to the head region, an area that is so complex and about which comparatively little is known, Therapeutic Touch should be done very gently. The hand should never be still, but constantly moving rhythmically, and, of course, the Therapeutic Touch practice should be done only for short periods of time.

The Throat Chakra

The physical focus for this field is approximately at the level of the medulla oblongata, at the base of the skull. Its vital-energy flow connects with the thyroid and the parathyroid glands, the former particularly concerned with the basic metabolism of the body (and therefore, important in wound healing). The throat chakra's general balance is also importantly affected in the building up and breaking down of cell tissue.

At the vital-energy level, the throat chakra is also concerned with the quality of space, the underlying basis of sound, and the medium of vibration. In reference to the first function, the appreciation of space, one aspect of Therapeutic Touch in this region might be to work with persons who are hemiplegic and have lost the ability to use the extremities on one side of their bodies due to brain injury. It also might be useful to include the throat chakra when working with athetoid cerebral-palsied children. With reference to this chakra's concern with sound, it is worth studying the effects of Therapeutic Touch on hearing impairments, and perhaps tinnitus, the neural damage that produces a constant ringing in the ears, Thirdly, since the throat chakra is sensitive to vibration, its use with persons who have speech impairments comes easily to mind.

The Heart Chakra

The heart chakra is related to an area midway between the shoulder blades. It is linked to the physical heart, the blood stream and its circulation, and the electrolytic balance of the lymphatics. The lymphatic system seems to balance the energies of the supraphysical by controlling the amount of blood flowing to any one area (Karagulla and Kunz, p. 93).

The heart chakra is the integrative center for the entire chakra system and, therefore, would be centrally involved in all states of illness or weakness of the physical body. It has a powerful relationship with the crown chakra and, in conjunction with it, is concerned with higher dimensions of consciousness; therefore, it is a major factor in spiritual transformation. It is a medium for the power and the quality of love, and thus can be importantly engaged during Therapeutic Touch practices with those who have been physically or psychologically abused or who are alienated. It can also be used judiciously in cases of resentment, hate, or jealousy. In these instances, the Therapeutic Touch therapist should engage the healee in the dynamic use of his or her own heart chakra, perhaps as a meditative practice. Meditation may also act to strengthen the heart chakra's connection to the core of the solar plexus chakra, and so bring stability and balance to the body's functions.

The heart chakra has the powerful attribute of motion, and, therefore, is useful in Therapeutic Touch practices with those who have problems with blood circulation or with circulation within the lymphatic system. Also, there is a significant relationship between the heart chakra and the thymus in the physical body. The thymus is a major component of the immunological system, and so should be considered in Therapeutic Touch practices for all infectious and disease states. In 1959, during an examination of the thymus, Dora Kunz reported perceiving the important role of the thymus in the immunological process. This was not found to be the case scientifically until 1960, and was not reported in professional journals until later in the 1960s. She also observed possible connections between the heart rhythm and emotional states, which then affected the thymus gland (p. 113).

The Solar Plexus Chakra

The solar plexus chakra is primarily related to the adrenal glands, the pancreas, liver, and stomach. Most significantly, it is the site where energies from the psychodynamic field enter the vital-energy field (p. 43). It is also closely related to the heart and the throat chakras. These chakras, therefore, are included as sites for Therapeutic Touch in instances of hyperactivity, in strong, uncontrolled emotions, such as rage and anger, and in psychosomatic illness. Therapeutic Touch practice in the solar plexus region can also be used for blood sugar (pancreas) and fluid and electrolytic (liver) imbalances, for digestive disorders, and in the healing of ulcerations in the gastrointestinal tract.

The Spleen Chakra

As noted, the spleen chakra is not considered a major chakra; however, it plays an important role in the chakra system. Physiologically its functions include the reforming of blood components, the storing of iron, and being a reservoir for red blood cells and a physiological filter for the immunological system. The spleen is one of the three most important sites for vital energy to enter the body. The other two are the skin and the lungs.

At the supraphysical level, the major function of the spleen is to absorb vitality (prana) from the vital-energy field, modify it, and then distribute it to the other chakras, thereby supplying them all with prana (pp. 43–44). Because of this critical ability to absorb and distribute prana, this site has significant functions in the practice of Therapeutic Touch, particularly for chronic fatigue syndrome, both preoperatively and in postoperative recuperation, and in times of crisis.

The Root Chakra

The root chakra lies at the base of the spine. As noted, it is the site of latent kundalini, and the site from which the major nadi, sushumna, accompanied by ida and pingala, arises. The sushumna, Dora Kunz observes, is concerned with the process of inflow of energies from the vital-energy field, whereas ida and pingala are involved with the process of outflow of these energies. Therefore, she points out, the root chakra is intrinsically associated with the life energies.

Through its special relationship with the crown chakra, the root chakra responds to the fundamental intentionality of the inner self (p. 45). Intentionality, of course, is central to the practice of Therapeutic Touch and, therefore, is responsive to this liaison.

The Psychodynamic Field

The seven chakras noted above in the vital-energy field have their counterparts in the psychodynamic field. These two fields do not have direct relations with any of the endocrine glands, except for the coccygeal body. Although this small gland was first described by anatomist George Luschkas in the nineteenth century, its function still is not understood. Dora Kunz has observed counterparts of the coccygeal body in all the fields of the personal self—that is, in the conceptual field as well as in the psychodynamic and the vital-energy fields. This relationship suggests that this site has more complex and important functions than we are presently aware of.

At the supraphysical level, she describes the root chakra as having an association with both the brain as an organ and with the pineal gland, and notes that it is especially correlated with the crown chakra, the coupling vivifying during certain states of consciousness (p. 121).

Because the fields at the level of the personal self are closely integrated, the effects at one level eddy into that of the next level, and thereby affect the associated structures as well. A specific description, as observed by Dora Kunz, is illustrative:

> ...emotions that are sustained over a long period of time remain fairly constant in the aura. If they are negative, such as depression or resentment, they can affect the flow of energy, and this has long-range effects in terms of the condition of the etheric (vital-energy field) and physical bodies. For example, states of anxiety appear as grayish-blue clouds within the astral (psychodynamic) field, localized toward the center of the body near the solar plexus chakra. This causes the astral energy to flow inward towards the body, inhibiting the normally free circulation of energy throughout the emotional field. The closer the gray-blue color is to the physical body, the more severe the degree of anxiety and the greater the degree of impact on health. When this color tends towards the periphery of the aura, this indicates that the subject is on the way to freeing himself from his anxiety. (p. 50)

Dora Kunz additionally points out that, in this way, each of us is "constantly creating waves and currents of emotional energy by the ways he responds to the world around him (for the). . . material of the astral world is very impressionable, and responds quickly to the thoughtforms or images which we imbue with our feelings" (p. 51).

She speaks specifically to those in the healing and helping professions, and cautions that, because of the strong linkages between the fields of the personal self, we must learn to keep our own sensitivities under control. It is possible, she says, to identify so strongly, consciously or unconsciously, with the feelings of other persons as to feel their pain or distress. In this way, we open ourselves by empathizing or taking in those feelings. She notes that if the causes are not understood, such persons ". . . may be considered hypochondriacs because the symptoms change constantly. . . . However, if it is controlled, it can become a valuable diagnostic tool" (p. 53).

The Conceptual Field

The conceptual field interpenetrates both the psychodynamic field and the vital-energy field. Dora Kunz notes that the conceptual field is finer grained and faster moving than the other two fields. It unites all avenues of consciousness and ". . . can both greatly affect disease processes and be a powerful force for health, growth and change." As with the chakras in the vital-energy field and their counterparts in the psychodynamic field, chakras at the level of the conceptual field are closely bound to their next higher frequency reflection (for example, *buddhic*, Skt.) at the intuitional level, the highest level of the personal self, which is available only under special conditions. This caveat is important to understand, for the bases of illness frequently go beyond the supraphysical, the psychodynamic, or the conceptual energy fields. The entire chakra system forms a closely knit and finely integrated network. Each chakra influences and is influenced by the other, even as the complex interacts as a totality, meanwhile evoking individual responses from the chakras. However, although it can be appreciated that the entire chakra system is very complex, it also must be recognized that it cannot be explicitly described with a high degree of validity, with reference only to three-dimensional frames.

Hints and Suggestions

Visualization

An astute observer can pick up several specific suggestions on, for instance, the importance of dynamically visualizing the intentionality of a healing. Therefore, as an extension of that insight, when having the healee use visualization to do "homework" as a method of reinforcing the healing being done by Therapeutic Touch, the therapist would have the healee visualize the assignment dynamically. The rationale for this approach is that if the image is rigidly held, it will have little effect on the living flow of the non-physical energy fields of the personal self (p. 63). To be most effective, visualization must be vitally energized. We realize, too, that it is very important, in assigning the visualization, to use a symbol or image that has some significance or inner meaning to the healee. Results of an experimental study that is cited by Dora Kunz concluded that, when visualization is purely a mental exercise, it does not seem to affect the chakras (p. 64). However, the chakras do respond to visualization of a symbol that has meaningful significance or relevance to the individual (p. 69). In this way, visualization can assist in the healing process for, in bringing the brow chakra into activity, it energizes the whole system, and this may have a useful effect upon the person's health (p. 169).

Meditation

Therapeutic Touch has been rightly called a walking meditation (Weber, 1986). Dora Kunz speaks to the importance of regularity for meditation to have the long-range effects of fostering a harmonic link between all levels of consciousness. Specifically, she says that meditation with regularity can alter repetitive behaviors that create tensions, even to significantly transforming the imprint of obnoxious personality traits. This will serve to improve the health of the individual as new energy flows to the chakras. In turn, this new flow affects the chakra's rhythms so that the chakras will again function in harmony. As this process goes into motion, it will further facilitate the individual's attempt to break destructive habit patterns.

Healers And Healing

Dora Kunz has observed that most people who use their hands for healing are using part of their own vital-energy fields to help the healee, although energies from the universal field are also involved in the healing process. Because of this, their vital-energy fields have more elasticity than those of the average person (Karagulla and Kunz, 1989, p. 93). She offers other wide-ranging hints. For instance, she has observed that synthetic materials, such as nylon and Dacron, partially inhibit the vital-energy flow, and she also has found the reverse to be true with natural materials, such as cotton, silk, and wool (p. 142). Sunlight, she observes, is very beneficial and increases vital energy, but exposure to the sun over long periods of time tends to deplete it. Studies with colored glass have demonstrated varying effects: When light shines through yellow or gold-colored glass, it energizes; blue light is soothing, reduces pain, and lowers blood pressure; green light has a harmonizing effect on the vital-energy field. Apparently, too, there are some differences produced by colored artificial light and the mental visualization of the same color. She also has observed that the form in which the color is used or visualized, for instance, a circle, triangle, or cross, may produce different effects (p. 143).

Descriptions at the Supraphysical Level

Various Stages of Recovery from Anesthesia

In studies on the effects of anesthesia, Dora Kunz has observed that when the anesthetized patient is unconscious, his or her vital-energy field appears to be pushed out of the body and hovers over the head. As the patient partially recovers, the vital-energy field begins to move down toward the trunk. Then, as the patient more fully recovers, there is a gradual return of the vital-energy field to the feet (p. 160).

Effects of Tranquilizers

In other studies, after a dose of Thorazine, the activities of the supraphysical brain slow down, as do the brow and throat chakras. The optic nerve, the hypothalamic region, and the pituitary gland are affected, and the mechanisms of both visual and auditory perceptions are dulled. After a half-hour, the tranquilizer has affected all three fields of the personal self, especially the psychodynamic, whose activities and functions are notably decreased (pp. 146–147).

Summary and Conclusions

Summarizing what we now know of the chakras as centers of consciousness, and the effects they have on health and disease, we find that they are stepped-down fields of different kinds of consciousness, which localize to form and to organize the human individual. At the level of the personal self, these include the conceptual, the psychodynamic, and the vital fields of human energy, and there also are localized fields of consciousness at the more spiritual levels. All of these localized fields interpenetrate and intimately and dynamically relate to one another at all levels of consciousness, so that an event in one affects the whole, even as the entire chakra complex significantly influences its several facets.

Sculpted out of these localized fields are vortices of human energy whose attributes lay the foundation for conscious awareness of objects, events, interactions, and relationships. Out of this complex, the mind coheres in the individual person. These fields of consciousness focus and feed their field energies to the individual through a network of supraphysical circuits, the nadis. As mentioned, the major nadis make contact with the person's nervous system and endocrine glands, and then affect the chemophysical and psychophysiological functioning. The fine integration and synchronization between the chakras themselves and within their several levels of organization in the conceptual, psychodynamic, and vital-energy fields, keep the individual in a healthy state. When dissonance, breaks in the energy field, or leakages of vital energy occur, the individual becomes vulnerable to illness and disease.

Seven of the major chakras are of particular importance to the practice of Therapeutic Touch, especially at the level of the vital-energy field. In response to specific changes in patterns of thinking and feeling, alteration in chakra dynamics is possible for the individual person; however, the attitude of the healee toward healing itself does not significantly affect the process. Therefore, a major goal of the Therapeutic Touch therapist is to help the healee in this understanding, and thereby facilitate the healee's access to self-healing.

There are other hints and suggestions for the Therapeutic Touch therapist to consider. Of prime importance is to seriously attempt to connect with the inner self, and in the process, learn experientially how the activities and functions of one's own chakra system play through the self. Although it is possible to do this for oneself, it is exceedingly difficult and, for most of us, impossible to structurally alter the dynamics of other persons' chakras. Each person must do that for him- or herself. However, we, as Therapeutic Touch therapists, can assist the vital-energy flows of the healee to work harmoniously toward the increase of vitality, the removal of blockages, the relief of pain, and other ways that support change of unhealthy states of behavior and enhance the healing process.

In particular, use of the heart chakra, in the therapist and the healee, is very helpful, since it is the center for the integration of the entire chakra complex. Through "homework" of visualizations, meditations, and other kinds of reinforcements, the healee can be taught an appreciation of heart chakra functions as part of the Therapeutic Touch session. The goal would be to bring his or her own abilities for self-healing to the fore by helping the healee to change psychosomatic patterns of behavior, repressions, and other emotional imbalances. In the session, meanwhile, the Therapeutic Touch therapist would be supporting the healee by directing, modulating, or unruffling the vital-energy flow with Therapeutic Touch practices.

Taking a hint from Dora Kunz's observations, in cases where there is infectious disease, the therapist can use the corresponding heart chakra area over the healee's thymus, at the base of the breastbone, to lend support to his or her immunological system. The heart chakra region is also a major focus for cardiac problems, and for circulatory, blood pressure, or fluid and electrolyte irregularities. Because of the heart chakra's unusual relationship to both the crown chakra and the sense of touch, doing Therapeutic Touch very gently and sensitively when persons are in final transition during the dying process, carries with it a sense of serenity. Application of this technique is also very helpful for persons who are in crisis or in great fear.

Working with the vital-energy flow in the region corresponding to the solar plexus chakra (over the sites of the adrenal glands) is particularly good with persons who are emotionally disturbed or who have psychosomatic symptoms. In our experience with Therapeutic Touch, we have consistently found that the vital-energy field over these sites is rapidly responsive in cases of extreme fatigue and for those recuperating from surgery or grave illness. Apparently it is a very safe procedure, for since our introduction of Therapeutic Touch—twenty-three years at this writing—we never have had reports of any untoward reactions to this Therapeutic Touch skill. In baffling cases, quiet meditation on the condition of the healee has been helpful to Therapeutic Touch therapists in clarifying how to proceed in the best interests of the ill person, and meditation also may lend insight into considerations of appropriate "homework" for the healee.

Working preventatively before an operation, many Therapeutic Touch therapists spend short periods of time during the preoperative week gently vitalizing the healee's energy field. This practice appears to be very stabilizing. After obtaining permission postoperatively from both the healee and any other appropriate sources, and while keeping a keen eye on the healee's vital signs and other psychophysiological signs while the healee is recovering from the anesthesia, a gentle unruffling of the vital-energy field is helpful in dissipating the anesthesia from the healee's system. In doing this, do not awaken him or her, for sleep is the body's most powerful regenerative ally. Be sensitive to your own heart chakra, and use it as a guide in creating a milieu of support and peace as you quietly do Therapeutic Touch. However, do Therapeutic Touch for only short periods of time until recovery from anesthesia is complete. At this stage the healee is usually conscious, and you can teach ventilatory exercises to help him or her to fully reoxygenate the lungs. If the healee is alert enough—or at another time—you can combine this with the exercise Explorations of the Self 3 (p. 13) to help this person more fully stabilize as the anesthetic gases continue to blow off.

For healees who are taking medications, such as tranquilizers or psychotropic drugs, it is important to work in the region related to the solar plexus chakra for the reasons suggested by Dora Kunz's observations, noted previously. Working in the vital-energy field related to the spleen chakra helps stimulate the uptake and distribution of prana. Also the liver handles several physiological functions that are important at this time, such as fluid and electrolyte balance. In the latter instance, concentrate efforts to support the entire physiological triad of the adrenal, thyroid, and pituitary glands. During the Therapeutic Touch assessment, search out a sense of breaks in the continuity of the vital-energy field, and then slowly and rhythmically unruffle the field, especially in the areas you noted need attention.

Since all three human energy fields of the personal self are drastically affected by these medications, you, as a person of conscience and as an advocate for the healee, can request moderating dosages of tranquilizers or psychotropic drugs. Frequently therapists from several allied modalities work as a team on a cooperative basis for the healee's benefit, and during treatment, support and keep in close contact with the healee. This combined effort provides excellent opportunities for re-educating the healee about his or her own health care and instilling an appreciation for the need of personal responsibility.

In Reflection

Therapeutic Touch, as a committed and compassionate practice, opens you to new insights, perspectives, and goals of both a personal and a professional nature. What is at stake in the practice of Therapeutic Touch is the opportunity to acquire a new consciousness. Once acquired, it is with fresh awareness that you consciously commit to learning, helping, and healing with the whole of your being, for you are the test object for the many personal effects of Therapeutic Touch practice.

In yearning toward this goal of personal insight, you easily, and often more effortlessly than could have been imagined, change both worldview and lifestyle. You become more sensitive to forces working from within as, for instance, an increasing awareness that a background of elegant universal laws subtly impinges upon and frames everyday life's activities. This is supported by a growing appreciation for precepts that guide inner evolution, but nevertheless guard individuals' rights to choose the unique path for their own lifeway. Over time these personal knowledges forge new perspectives from which to view the mystery that underlies the healing process. You then begin to realize that personal engagement with the Therapeutic Touch process can evoke subtle transformations in the very being of the individual, so that its practice becomes an art form, and in the expression of this art, your muse, you find, is the deep, inner self.

Why do I want to be healer? In search of the muse, I know.

PRANA: THE ENERGY THAT HELPS US HEAL

The Notion of Human Energy

"B'golly, the blinkin' foot has gone numb!" I exclaimed while stamping my foot at the side of the old swimming hole. It was the first day of a Therapeutic Touch workshop that Dora Kunz and I were doing together, and a very hot one, the temperature hovering near 100 degrees and the low barometric pressure promising a thunderstorm.

I had finished my morning classes and, because of the oppressive weather, I decided to take a swim instead of going to lunch. I had whistled up my dogs, hurried down to the swimming hole, and waded out, anticipating the refreshing plunge when the waters got deep enough. Hip-deep into the water, I noticed that a workshop participant was standing at the edge of the swimming hole, waving and calling my name. I turned around to face her and found myself engaged in a half-hour discussion.

Finally she left and I dove into the water for a quick swim. It was as I was climbing the bank of the swimming hole that I noticed what I thought were numbing sensations in my right leg. My concern was heightened because the leg had been operated on several months before for a congenital anomaly in the bone structure. In an attempt to save me from a more extensive operation, the surgeon had revised part of the knee joint and had retailored the tibia. However, severe nerve damage had resulted, with intense, constant pain throughout the entire leg.

In a series of intensive Therapeutic Touch sessions over a three-day period, Dora Kunz had been able to eradicate the pain in the upper leg to just below the knee. Over the next six months by doing Therapeutic Touch to myself, I had been able to reduce the pain in my lower leg to about ankle level. However, the nerves in the sole of my foot continued to be so sensitive that it took me a few minutes of exercise each morning before I could bear to stand on them. There continued to be minimal discomfort as I walked, but I had gotten used to that. Now, as I came out of the water, my constant companion seemed gone; no pain, not even a bit.

I walked up to my cabin, still thinking that my leg was simply numbed by standing waist-deep in the cold stream for a half-hour. Later, however, even though I stamped my foot frequently as I walked down to rejoin the workshop group, the pain did not return. Since the workshops would continue for two weeks, I decided not to say anything about it, but to observe the leg carefully during that time.

The leg continued to function well and was pain-free. At the end of the workshop, Dora and I were sitting out on the lawn answering last-minute questions. Finally, all had gone and I told Dora about the incident and asked her what she thought had happened. She looked at my leg and then said, "You know, we do not realize how much prana there is in fresh running water." I had not been thinking about a miracle, but the simple truth of what she said startled me. Yes, I realized, we do not appreciate the abundance of vital energies around us in the living waters, the respiring trees, the ever-present, life-giving sun whose outpouring of prana is vital to the fundamental functionings of our entire solar system. Prana, the energy that constantly flows through us to keep us vital and healthy and, when necessary, to help us to heal; this wonderous mystery, all around us, but so little noticed or appreciated.

Prana underlies the organization of what we call the "life process," and sustains all breathing creatures (Avalon, p. 74). Its functions of vitalizing and providing cohesion to the matter of the physical body are derived from the universal force, *Vayu* (*va*, Skt.: to move; for example, rhythmically). As noted in chapter 4, the incessant upwelling of pranic flow is individually tailored to each person through her or his chakras. This pranic flow makes itself known by its masterly organization of fundamental cyclic life forces; when movement stops, life stops.

Prana is a complex of subsystems, five of which are assimilable by the human body at this time in our evolution. We cannot observe the difference between the living and the nonliving without realizing that all life forms differentiate their signs of aliveness, such as vitality or pranic flow, by functions which reflect an underlying ordered rhythmicity of movement that is closely coupled with an exquisite timing of function. Rhythmicity can be perceived in even the most fundamental forms of respiration, pulsation, and coordinated movement. An example of the combination of the last two factors is the peristalsis of the gut, which moves solid waste products out of the body; and an illustration of the integration of all three factors is the in- and out-breathing of the lungs as they blow off the waste products of respiration.

The Silent Mantra

The inhalation-exhalation cycle itself is said to be a mantra that "is not recited, for it is said without volition" (p. 77). It operates independent of our waking consciousness, and its self-regulating processes function from a subconscious level that only occasionally is required to submit to conscious will. Therefore, it is said that prana does not do its work at the level of the inhalation and exhalation, but at the level of the underlying dynamism. Even at the molecular level that undergirds the pulsing waves of peristalsis, a metered cadence of forces of the metabolic processes function within the microtissues of the gut. Also, rhythmicity marks the cellular base of the respiratory process itself. In the bloodstream, we find the measured, rhythmic deposition of oxygen molecules twinned to the simultaneous uptake of molecules of carbon dioxide as the bloodstream floods each cell, providing it with fresh oxygen to carry on the critical functions of the oxidation process that fuels the body's functions. The incessant beating of the heart, the cyclic emptying of the gallbladder, and the functions of the entire genitourinary system are but an additional few of the countless examples of physiological rhythmicity. Indeed, we find this characteristic signature of explicit timing resonating throughout the human body as it goes about its daily activities of living.

It is this pervasive statement of primal rhythmic movement (to-fro, in-out, particle-wave) that forms the background for the momentary states of balance toward which the Therapeutic Touch therapist strives to assist the healee through the projection of healing energies. One of the clues that hints at this rhythmicity is mirrored in the Therapeutic Touch process itself. Whenever two therapists simultaneously work on a healee, although they may do their assessments of the healee's condition separately, at their individual pace, they have to finely coordinate their acts of rebalancing for the healing to significantly benefit the healee. In fact, if they are not in synch, they may adversely affect the healee. To an observer watching this rhythmic interplay between the healers, it is as though a gentle, elegant pavane was being danced within the delicate gossamer of the healee's vital-energy field. As the healee begins to respond to this compassionate yet graceful enactment of healing, he or she is joined to the dance in a further act of grace.

The Stream of Vital Energies

As has been discussed in chapter 4, human energies flow from the chakras and are subject to their influence. These vital forces are channeled within the individual's vital-energy field through the nadis. The nadis are thought to be 72,000 in number, and they act as miniducts or energyways to convey the pranic flows. They have been likened to the minute networks of fibers that conduct nutrients throughout the leaves of trees. It is said that as prana runs through the nadis, it acts as a conveyor for *citta.* Citta is the aspect of our perceptions that puts us in contact with the environment through sensory input.

In rough translation, it can be said that the essential elements of prana stream through the splenic chakra of the individual, where five of its seven subsystems are converted into assimilable form and distributed in various combinations of the subsystems through the nadis. These units or sets vitalize the major organs and tissues of the body. When this process is completed, these units of prana flow and meet in the vital-energy field in the region between the two shoulder blades, at the confluence of the brachial plexus. They then stream down the nonphysical vital-energy complement of the arms to what is termed "the knot" (granthis) of the wrist. The pranic streams are reconstituted to their original five subsystems, and the subsystems of prana exit, each through one of the five fingers.

The Subsystems of Prana

Although the functions somewhat overlap, exact specialization of dynamic and vitalizing functions apportioned to each subsystem is known (see figure 6). Recognizing that prana is a universal force, the functions of its five subsystems are individually defined.

The first subsystem is also called prana and it is said to reside in the region of the heart, in a place called "The Abode of the Mother." It is the subtle energy complex that fundamentally supports the life process; for instance, as noted, the subsystem prana forces us to inhale. Western physiology tells us that automatic inhalation is driven by the difference in pressure gradients in the lungs after exhalation. However, what is pressure other than "the exertion of continuous force on a unit area," and in the present context, the substratum of this "continuous force" has a name—prana—with a few additionally perceived characteristics.

The second subsystem is called *udana.* Its sphere of responsibility is the region of the throat, and it causes the upward movement of

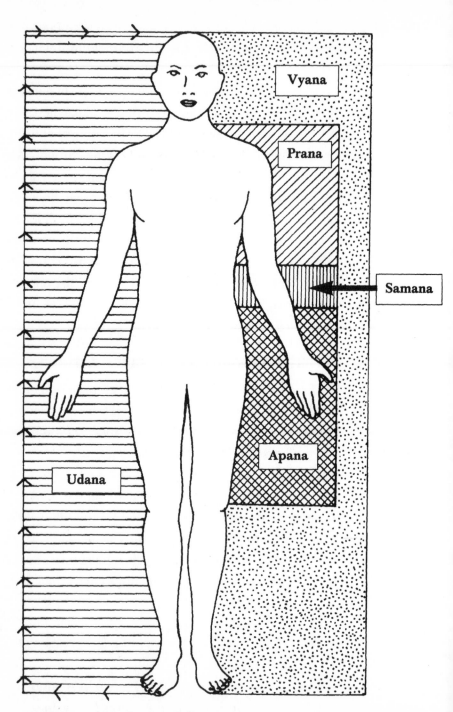

FIGURE 6: Subsystems of Prana

exhalation. By the use of the mind, udana enables speech and evokes power in the form of sound, called "mantra" (from the Sanskrit root, *man*, to think). The third subsystem is *apana*. Apana localizes in the region of the lower bowels, in the domain of the mulhadhara chakra. Avalon calls it the downward "breath" that pulls against prana, and presses downward. It causes various secretory flows and governs the major excretory functions of the body.

Samana, the fourth subsystem, is at the umbilicus, in the region of the solar plexus chakra. It is called "the fire that equalizes everything," which appears to refer to the process of oxygenation by which the basic metabolic functions of the body are carried on. Samana "kindles the bodily fire" and regulates the faculties of assimilation, digestion, and respiration. The fifth subsystem is *vyana*, which penetrates the entire body and resists the powers of disintegration. Vyana provides the forces of cohesion at the molecular level so that the body and its parts are held together. It is thought to cause muscular movement (and even movement within muscular tissue itself, as in the ripple effect of smooth muscle tissue). It is also involved in the circulation of blood and in metabolic functions. In addition, there are minor aspects or minisystems that are mentioned that are concerned with deep-seated reflexes, such as yawning, hiccoughing, and opening and closing of the eyes (p. 78).

Prana, through its subsystems, permeates all activities by which we define life. It quickens and infuses all creatures with the vitality, vigor, and vivacity that mark aliveness and well-being. History and tradition verify that the human being, who, as science agrees, is the only creature able to voluntarily control vital functions such as breathing, can also transfer his or her underlying dynamic—prana—to another person. One technique for doing this is through controlled breathing. Other techniques include using the eye gaze, making certain movements of the hand, and through intentionality. The last two are acknowledged tools of Therapeutic Touch. I would like to explore how breathing also may be counted as an ally of the Therapeutic Touch interaction.

How Therapeutic Touch Uses the Subsystems Of Prana

Fundamentally, the Therapeutic Touch therapist tries to repattern, rebalance, or knit together the healee's vital-energy field so that he or she can function again as an integral whole. How this occurs is a mystery to many—as much a mystery as the internal processes of other healing modalities. However, the therapist easily recognizes while working with Therapeutic Touch that the potency of centering the consciousness, when it is done competently as an interior act, is the undeniable source of power.

It looks quite simple to the observer and seems so to the beginner; however, mature centering of the consciousness is, in fact, a complex act of conscious exploration of the inner self. Over time, the psychophysiological effects of the centering act are profound. Centering is then characterized by:

- Psychomotor quieting and a sense of inner equilibrium
- Significant lessening of the monkey chatter of the brain
- Sense of timelessness
- Lessening of egocentric focus
- Significant increase in the simultaneity of life experiences
- Change of worldview
- Consequent change in lifestyle
- Clarity in the recognition of compassion as power
- Deepening appreciation of conscious mindfulness
- Stronger grasp of intuitive insights
- Access to deep inquiry
- Tacit understanding of effortless effort

The therapist remains on-center throughout the entirety of the Therapeutic Touch interaction, even as he or she also goes on to the other phases of the process. Needing to understand what is the matter with the healee, the therapist does an assessment of the healee's vital-energy field. The nature of the vital-energy field presents itself basically in a perceived on-off display; that is, the field is sensed, primarily through the hand chakras, as being in a state of either balance or imbalance. As with pregnancy, there does not seem to be an intermediate state, although various background qualifiers can be sensed as additional cues. In general, therefore, the nature of the healee's vital-energy field presents itself bimodally to the healer as either having a free flow or as being overlaid by a sense of congestion or sluggishness; there is either a rhythmic or a dysrhythmic pulsing to the flow. The structure of the field seems to have pattern or the configurations within it are random and ragged, so that overall there is either a perception of balance, dynamic equilibrium, and order, or a sense of unevenness, imbalance, and instability.

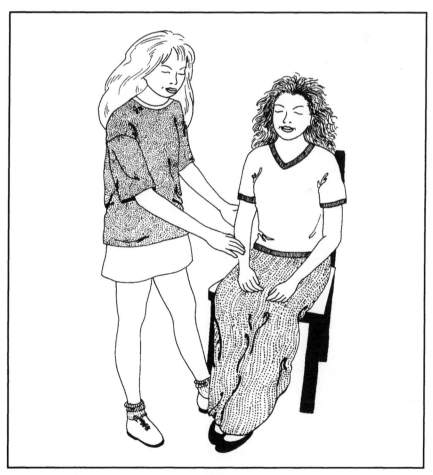

FIGURE 7: Therapeutic Touch therapist and healee

The Constancy of Vital-Energy-Field Cues

Throughout the long 15,000-year history of the therapeutic use of hands, there has been an awesome constancy in the descriptors healers have used to specify what they sense in the healee's vital-energy field, cues that indicate that the healee is ill. This amazing agreement in the choice of descriptors has also held true over the past quarter century for Therapeutic Touch therapists' descriptions of the cues they sense in the healee's vital-energy field while they are doing an assessment (Krieger, 1993, p. 31). These descriptors or cues of imbalance have been derived subjectively; however, they do lend themselves to broad categorization into five general groupings. Moreover, within each group, the cues appear to relate to a common level of experience or consciousness. From this perspective, these cues present themselves in the following sets:

1. Cues related to temperature differentials are the most frequently sensed. These are concerned with sensations of heat, cold, or a variation that is described as a "hollow" coldness that seems to flow out of a vacuum. This level of consciousness most frequently entails an explicit awareness of a significant difference of temperature in a clearly demarcated region of the healee's vital-energy field.

2. Another common description is that of a magnetic pulling or drawing of the hand to a particular site in the healee's vital-energy field. This movement appears to happen without the healer's volitional control, the hand automatically shifting to a specific area, which is then recognized as being out of balance to the rest of the field. While this is occurring, the healer seems to be involved with an interior evaluation processing of the perceptions of the hand chakras and perhaps other factors unknown at this time. Descriptors such as "congestion" or "fullness" are also perceived at this level of consciousness.

3. A third level of consciousness is concerned with frank metaphors, variously described as "tinglings," "little electric shocks," "burstings of little bubbles," or as "pins and needles." These cues seem more imbued with the individual expression of the healer, but all respond to a common method of rebalancing, which is to dampen the cue through an induction of the relaxation response, or a quiet, firm "unruffling" of the vital-energy field to "even" out the area.

4. The sensing of rhythmic pulsations of the vital-energy field is a cue that is less often perceived. Subjectively, dysrhythmias seem to have a distinct relationship to the chakras of the healee, and may be involved in the illness.

5. Deep insights into the healee's condition that are truly intuitive indicate a fifth level of consciousness. These cues are least frequent, but have a high reliability. This state is perceived as a distinct shift from everyday consciousness.

The assignment of levels to these experiences is arbitary. At first these descriptors seemed to be only interesting, and I treated them in a straightforward manner. I gathered these data from Therapeutic Touch therapists as they worked with their clients, and I assigned categories according to simple, gross characteristics. These preliminary groupings were then examined for indications of underlying sets according to simple variables, such as cues that were easily discerned early in the Therapeutic Touch experience of the therapist (for instance, temperature differential and magnetic pull). Other cues included those that seemed to convey similar meanings to the therapist, such as "tinglings" or "bubbles"; those that seemed to require a long period of experience to access, such as the rhythmic-dysrhythmic spectrum; and those that were rare and seemed to require a sensitivity that depended on personal practices by the Therapeutic Touch therapist, such as true intuitive insight into the healee's problems. With additional experience with Therapeutic Touch, most therapists can relate to more than one level with ease—for example, picking up temperature differential cues in one area of the healee's field and "tingle" in another. Others can relate to more than two levels and, rarely, a few can relate to all five levels. Where a therapist can relate to more than one level, it appears that one or two levels predominate during the course of an individual assessment.

Cues as Communication

As noted previously, the name given the cue by the Therapeutic Touch therapist seems to be a metaphor that is not applicable literally—for instance, the temperature differentials. Nevertheless, the cues can convey specific meaning to another Therapeutic Touch therapist. When so engaged, we realize that there are other means of communication apparently taking place about events that are non-physical, and that the communication has a personal validity that is as equally as subtle as the vital-energy structures with which they deal. At this time in seventy-five countries of the world Therapeutic Touch appears to be a natural transcultural human potential that can be realized under appropriate circumstances. We come to the realization that this sensitivity, which is so central to the Therapeutic Touch experience, also might be considered a natural potential and, therefore, the Therapeutic Touch assessment could be accessed and described as a subjective reality common to most people.

Foundations for Hypothesis

The following are the major points made about how the vital-energy field is used in the Therapeutic Touch process:

- We know what the vital-energy flows feel like.
- They appear to constellate into patterns.
- Therapists can sense these patterns as cues to the balanced or unbalanced condition of the healee's vital-energy field.
- The vital-energies have several levels of organization.
- Therapeutic Touch therapists of some experience can communicate information about these vital energies to one another

with a high degree of reliability.

- They can knowledgeably modulate, modify, shift, and transform these cues—for instance, change a cue of congestion or sluggishness to one of free flow. As a result, in a large percentage of cases the healee's vital-energy flows are rebalanced, the symptoms abate, and the healee reports an alleviation of the condition and a sense of well-being.

Lama A. Govinda, a renowned scholar of Tibetan Buddhism, notes that the hand chakras, which are the tools of trade of the Therapeutic Touch therapist, are "important centers of psychic energy . . . second only to the major centers in the brain, throat, heart, navel, and reproductive organs" (Govinda, p. 55). Having noted that hand movements express attitude and, therefore, can be "spontaneous expressions of our deeper consciousness," he goes on to say that when a person engages in the therapeutic use of hands, the successive positions of the hands assume gestures that often symbolize inner experiences or spiritual attitudes that are taking place in the deeper consciousness, behaviors that may be beyond the person's everyday awareness. Such gestures are called *mudras* (Skt.). Mudras have the ability to guide, if not control, the universal force, prana, within the individual's vital-energy field. It can be assumed that these phenomena also occur in the Therapeutic Touch interaction, particularly if it is done with an intentionality embedded in knowledge and guided by compassion.

When the Therapeutic Touch interaction is viewed in the context of basic assumptions of contemporary physiology, we know that the human being is the only terrestrial being to have volitional control over certain vital functions. When that knowledge is coupled to the premises of Govinda that these vital functions are fundamentally based in pranic flows (which have originated from the five primary subsystems of the universal force, prana), and to the fact that human beings have the ability to transfer prana to another person, what can we add that would clarify how healing occurs during the Therapeutic Touch process?

We can acknowledge that it is the act of centering in the deep consciousness and the continuation of that state of consciousness throughout the process that is the source of empowerment during the Therapeutic Touch interaction. For the Therapeutic Touch therapist, the conscious enactment of the process itself forces the recognition that during the assessment phase there is a direct experience of the healee's vital-energy field. The condition of the healee's field presents itself to the hand chakras, which are interpreted by the therapist through a spectrum of subjective cues. These cues can be grouped according to the therapist's expertise, extent of practice, and/or sensitivity to subtle human energies. There is also the perception that the positioning of the hands (and the body in relation to them) during the rebalancing or healing process can be regarded as mudras, which symbolize inner experiences and spiritual attitudes that are occurring spontaneously in the deep consciousness of the Therapeutic Touch therapist. We also know that the rebalancing is guided by a decided intentionality. Intentionality implies that this healing act is firmly directed not only by the will of the therapist who wants the healee to get better, but also by the therapist's goal for the healee's recovery. This goal is based in the personal knowledge about the healee's condition that was acquired during the Therapeutic Touch assessment.

Healing as Metaneed

These dynamic processes have stemmed from the Therapeutic Touch therapist's initial expression of compassion for the suffering of the healee. Compassion is a sincere, deeply sympathetic passion to help or to heal, an intense, selfless concern about someone who is ill, in pain, or otherwise suffering. The power inherent in the compassionate impulse can be awesome. Later, people are amazed by the immensity of physical effort they could call upon to meet the exigencies of the situation, or the profound spiritual values they could call up from inner deeps. Expressions of compassion arise out of a "need-to-help" or a "need-to-heal", which, it seems to me, are second-order- or metaneeds, a concept introduced by the psychologist, Abraham Maslow. Maslow's development of a human needs theory convinced him of the crucial importance of metaneeds to the well-being of the psyche. This led him to conclude that without the expression of metaneeds in one's life ". . . the soul will surely die." Within a conceptual framework of the need-to-heal as a metaneed, history has revealed that the moral nature of the quasi-healer unable or unwilling to follow the guidance of the compassionate impulse also withers and deteriorates.

In contrast, what we find for the healers who follow the upwelling urge to help or to heal those in need, is that forces born in the compassionate act become allies, in both the working through of the situation that gave expression to the compassion and in the strengthening of the finespun ties to their inner selves. Therapists attest that the spontaneous, irresistible forces of compassion frequently carry us to states of consciousness, or at least to glimpses of these states, as they have been described by mystics in the past. When we examine the list of characteristics of the act of centering by the accomplished Therapeutic Touch therapist, one of the indicators is an increase in the understanding of compassion as power, and the stages that may follow are similar to the time-honored goals of the mystic and the philosopher.

Hypothesis of the Healing Silent Mantra

We can now begin to plot out hypothetical suppositions that may act as ground for further, more formal, investigations into the Therapeutic Touch interaction. To follow along with the development of this schema, I suggest that you use a copy of the "Deep Dee" outline (see p. 18) on which you have recorded the processing of your own Therapeutic Touch interactions. Using the "Deep Dee" to refresh your memory of the event, see whether the following suggestions for developing a working hypothesis about how the Therapeutic Touch therapist processes subtle human energies to help or to heal coincides with your own experience, and add your commentaries. It should be noted that in bringing these dynamic interactions under closer scrutiny, we will grapple with the details in a series of phases. In doing so, the timing of these events will be slowed down. Although it is the nature of several of these factors to occur simultaneously, in fact, during the Therapeutic Touch process, time itself does not conform to our usual conceptions.

In the beginning there is the upwelling urge of compassion that is experienced by the Therapeutic Touch therapist. The dynamics of this powerful, humane expression serve to heighten sensitivity to the healee. Centering into the deep consciousness so that you can become more aware of the stability of your own inner self, you begin the assessment. In doing so, you become more acutely sensitive to cues that indicate the nature of the vital-energy flows throughout the healee's field. You are now in a "listening" attitude, maintaining a quiet, but alert state of awareness to the cues in the healee's vital-energy field, and a keen-edged sensitivity to nuances that indicate the healee as a total individual, in his or her fullness of expression.

As your hand chakras seek out cues, you frequently engage in inner dialogue as you question yourself about your findings, or recognize relationships between factors in the vital-energy field, or wonder, "What else?" Concluding your assessment and still on- center, you decide how you will go about rebalancing the vital-energy flows in the healee's field, and then deploy these techniques. At a time deemed appropriate to the situation, you reassess the healee's vital-energy field to be assured of the integrity of the vital-energy flows and that the field is in fact balanced.

To shift perspective slightly, once more we will begin with the initial rush of compassion that proceeds the Therapeutic Touch interaction. Compassion, as previously noted, is essentially a passion for another's well-being. The concerned person is fully present to the healee, and the power of compassion acts to integrate the healer's efforts on behalf of the healee. A ripple effect of this potent surge reinforces the therapist's confidence and determination to help the healee. Compassion is a positive act. It is accompanied by an unwavering certainty that the therapist must act to meet the needs of the healee. This assurance, joined to the strong desire to help, serves to integrate the Therapeutic Touch therapist's actions.

When the therapist centers, there is a quieting of psychomotor activities, and an equilibrium is felt as a delicate sense of a pervasive inner balance. This provides a fine-tuned sounding board against which the grosser imbalances in the healee's vital-energy field stand out sharply as the therapist evaluates the healee's status. The act of centering also serves to coordinate facets of the therapist's deeper consciousness and, as these aspects of the inner self are called upon, the therapist has the opportunity to realize previously unheeded potentials to help or to heal.

The Therapeutic Touch assessment is a direct experience of the healee's vital-energy field and acts as a source for personal knowledge about it. The quality of this relationship deepens over time. The heightened awareness provided by the centering experience serves as a discriminative monitoring background to differentiate and characterize the cues as they are intercepted by the hand chakras. This personally codified information acts as a base for perceived connections between cues and other factors relating to the healee's condition, and ideas for therapeutic intervention, suppositions, and suggestions. Out of this compendium of perceptions, the therapist will draw up a plan for the rebalancing of the healee's vital-energy field.

The rebalancing phase itself is marked by a background of focused concentration and sensitive visualization as the Therapeutic Touch therapist attempts to follow the promptings accessed by the centered deep consciousness. This phase may include positionings of the hands in new or novel gestures. There is a decided but just perceptible moment when the therapist knows that the cue is in balance again. The Therapeutic Touch reassessment itself is a recap of known territory, to evaluate whether the cue being worked on is still activated (indicating that the vital-energy field is not in balance yet), if the rebalancing has accomplished what the therapist had anticipated, and if the healee's vital-energy flows have adequately resumed. The assessment also checks other aspects of the interaction whose relationship or meaning may now be more apparent to the therapist.

To add a final dimension to this investigation, consider one of the prime physiological functions that underlies these integrated activities of body, emotions, mind, and aspiration: breathing. Breathing, of course, accompanies all of the above-noted interactive factors; however, its very ubiquity may be why we overlook its possible importance to crucial functions of the Therapeutic Touch process. The physical positioning of the body and its extremities, the emotional involvement in the moment, the mental control that follows in the wake of intentionality, the archetypal behaviors that are called forth by the insistent urges to compassionate response, all affect the intrinsic rhythm, depth, and metabolic flow of the act of breathing.

Simply said, the various phases of Therapeutic Touch cause the therapist to use his or her breath in different ways to reinforce the expressions of these therapeutic engagements: a shift in breathing pattern as he or she centers; a short holding of the breath, and then a continued breathing rate that is barely perceptible as incoming data is focussed on; and a simultaneous use of breath to recruit, direct, or modulate the appropriate forces to rebalance the healee's vital-energy field. The enfolding intentionality also affects the breathing, we might say, subvocally. The breathing patterns that accompany each of the phases of Therapeutic Touch cause the inhaled air to exert a variable pressure on the soft tissues of the oral cavity and the esophageal tract and their underlying neural and circulatory nets. By such means, the flows of the pranic subsystems that accompany these anatomical structures are also significantly affected, and the whole synergistically reinforces the energetic effects of the mudralike gestures embedded in the Therapeutic Touch process.

It is said that the breath and the mind act upon one another. Reflecting back to Govinda's statement that breathing has been called the "silent mantra," we could posit an analogue between the effect of breathing during the Therapeutic Touch interaction in its full form and the effect of breathing during the sounding of a mantra.

The conception of mantra includes the notion of an irresistible drive to express a mental image, so that a mantra is a tool by which a mental picture is created, giving a reality to the intentionality of the mantra. Can we conjecture that the clear visualization of the non-physical interaction that plays an important role in Therapeutic Touch is similarly aroused by the breathing pattern (accompanied by the mind) of the Therapeutic Touch therapist? As with the mantra, the outflowing energies are closed off or redirected under the compelling forces of the intentionality and the vivid visualizations that accompany it, both of which are being utilized by the therapist to reinforce the directing or modulating of vital energies. Thus, in the act of turning inward, the silent mantra of the therapist's breathing patterns transforms into inaudible vibration. In ancient texts on mantra yoga, this inner vibration is said to have a resonating effect on the subsystems of prana, which in this case are acting as an integrated whole on behalf of the healee. It is further said that for this enactment of healing to be fully expressed, it must first be realized in the depth of the human heart. Thus, compassion can be seen as an ally; it is in the compassion that underlies the need-to-heal of the Therapeutic Touch therapist that this realization is enabled to transform into the vibrant, living force that is both healing and life-affirmative. When this is the setting for the Therapeutic Touch interaction, no magic is needed for the scenarios described above to be touched with reality.

Summary

A conceptual frame within which the underlying dynamism of the Therapeutic Touch process can be examined perceives prana as the foundational energetic that vivifies all living beings. Prana works through the individual as a complex of five subsystems of vital flow, whose major underlying characteristic is rhythmic motion. In the human being, these vital energies flow through energyways to circulate and distribute combinations of these subsystems of prana, each of which has specialized functions.

Human beings are the only terrestrial creatures who can control certain vital functions, such as breathing, and who can volitionally transfer prana to another being. Therapeutic Touch is one way that prana can be so transmitted. The source of power in Therapeutic Touch is the act of centering the consciousness, a state which continues throughout the entire Therapeutic Touch interaction. Therapeu-tic Touch is an act of conscious exploration by the therapist of aspects of his or her inner self. The enactment of centering as a worldview and subsequent lifestyle has several definable characteristics.

The Therapeutic Touch assessment is a conscious, direct experience of the healee's vital-energy field. Therapeutic Touch therapists maintain a consistency of description of their individual, subjective assessments of imbalances in the vital-energy fields of healees, and can communicate the validity of this information to each other. These descriptors, or cues, can be categorized into groupings that have relationships to the length of experience with Therapeutic Touch practice and/or the sensitivity of the Therapeutic Touch therapist. For instance, the therapist may relate to one level of perception, or may be able to access several levels. In Therapeutic Touch the hand chakras are major centers of consciousness. The hand gestures can act as mudras when they are positioned with intentionality, and sensitively symbolize inner experiences and spiritual attitudes. Mudras have the ability to guide and control prana. These dynamic processes are set in motion by the initial expression of compassion for the suffering of the healee, and act to further empower the healer's efforts to help or to heal.

During the Therapeutic Touch interaction, the therapist often engages in inner dialogue as the healee's condition is evaluated. He or she decides upon the strategies to be used, and then permits the perceptions that arise from a deeper consciousness to integrate themselves into conscious evaluations. The subsequent rebalancing of the healee's vital-energy field includes important positionings of the hands that may be new or novel to the therapist, different from the manner in which he or she uses them in everyday activities. These gestures, which rhythmically and smoothly follow one another through the Therapeutic Touch process, may be considered to have features similar to mudras.

The mudralike gestures that are being positioned with intentionality during the Therapeutic Touch interaction are reinforced by breathing patterns that accompany the therapist's focus of concentration to direct or modulate the flows of the pranic subsystems. They are also coupled with breathing patterns that express the therapist's attitudes and the intentionality itself.

Breathing can be considered a "silent mantra." During the Therapeutic Touch interaction, under the influence of the upsurging press of compassion and the firm commitment of intentionality, breathing patterns reinforced by the mudralike gestures serve to channel the flow of the active pranic subsystems, directing and modulating expressions of the Therapeutic Touch process that are being performed to help or to heal someone in need.

One More Word

As noted, these are but musings and speculations, at best a conceptual framework limited by a circumscribed ability to conceive. Nevertheless, they arise out of valid personal experience with nonphysical processes that do tweak the mind.

These wonderings will need objective confirmation for public acceptance. Such verification calls for a new kind of research. And who will answer that call? Obviously the needs of this "hi-touch" inquiry are diametrically opposed to "hi-tech" research design and methodologies, necessitating a different perception. However, one of the boons for the insightful pioneer who can meet such stringent standards will be a further glimpse into the wellsprings of the query: *Why do I want to be healer?*

THERAPEUTIC TOUCH AS A DIFFERENT KIND OF INTELLIGENCE

The Persistent Reality

There is a strange phenomenon that may occur in the lives of those who study in depth the effects of various modes of healing. It frequently happens that, after the researcher's studies have demonstrated the validity of the healing (as a therapeutic mode distinct from allopathic, traditional medicine), the researcher often reports a personal need to learn how to heal. The persistence of the reality of human ability to help presses upon the researcher with an unusual urgency. It is not a far flight of fancy to recognize that this curious occurrence appears to act in opposition to a principle well known in physics, Heisenberg's principle of complementarity. Heisenberg's principle states that scientists' observations in themselves are enough to change the phenomenon being studied. The strangeness is that the opposite effect happens in reference to healing. When the researcher studies this phenomenon—healing—it changes the researcher. This frequently results in a significant transformation in the researcher's lifestyle as experiences in helping or healing others deepen.

Healing as a lifestyle is not a miracle way; it's hard work. The conviction that healing others is a natural potential, which I firmly believe, does not minimize the fact that this potential can be realized only in a climate that nourishes the basic needs of others. To remain healthy in such a demanding environment, the healer must couple that consideration for others with a wholesome recognition of his or her own needs. Within this matrix of concern the healer demonstrates a commitment to healing, and her or his lifestyle is thereby declared. However, it is only in the working through of that self-asserted obligation that we begin to capture a clear notion of the immensity of changes that are entailed with the declaration to this persistent reality.

Therapeutic Touch: A Living Matrix of Inner Work

Therapeutic Touch is a contemporary interpretation of several ancient healing practices. At the minimum these venerable therapeutic skills integrate:

1. the continued centering of the healer's consciousness as a backdrop to the Therapeutic Touch process itself

2. some aspects of the laying-on of hands

3. the therapeutic use of the vital-energy field

4. visualization

5. the knowledgeable use of the therapist's own chakras

6. the use of breath in the expression of intentionality

7. the expression of compassion as power

8. mind-to-mind communication, particularly for those who are in critical condition, near death, or unable to communicate; it is also helpful for children and persons who are psychotic.

Many processes seem to be involved. How do they come together into a coherent whole? The answer is: very naturally. As a culture we have such a compulsion to categorize that, even though we experience continuity, we have conditioned ourselves to think in bits and bytes. Let us look at the actual process. Imagine that I am doing a Therapeutic Touch session with someone who is ill, and I am describing to you my inner work as I strive to help or to heal. I will demonstrate that, at the least, the above-noted techniques are integrated as they are needed, as the healee and I work toward a goal of well-being. As previously noted, however, although I will cite the skills one after another, you will appreciate that some aspects of this inner work are occurring simultaneously. With this in mind, then, to begin the Therapeutic Touch interaction:

1. I am centered. I feel profoundly quiet within and in a protected and permissive place.

2. I really want to help this person, and I can. To do this I have to smoothly and skillfully focus the many facets of my being, maintain that unified state, and, with a singleness of purpose, use this effortlessly balanced turning point as a fulcrum for incisive power during this act of healing.

3. I align myself with an aspiration to help or to heal this person, and I allow the flow of this persistent drive to course through me to the healee.

4. I recognize the rhythmic pulse of that pranic streaming and use my breath to bind with intentionality selected vital-energy flows.

5. As I work, I visualize the directing and modulating of vital energies to meet the needs of the healee.

6. I access my own chakras, and am sensitive to their various components of consciousness.

7. This transfer of vital pranic flow is reinforced by a surge of compassion that I have directed toward the healee. This humane outpouring of personal concern also acts as a medium for emotional support, encouragement, and reassurance to the healee as we communicate mind-to-mind.

8. I convey these thoughts with specific intentionality; the healee recognizes them, and in an expression of relief, he or she often verbalizes something such as, "I've never been touched in this way before," and opens him- or herself to healing as my inner work continues.

As noted above, these eight ancient healing practices are only some of those used in the practice of Therapeutic Touch. However, without a doubt, the power of Therapeutic Touch arises out of the centering of consciousness. In fact, this background state of consciousness is the imprimatur of Therapeutic Touch and is the unique contribution that Therapeutic Touch has made to society. It is the source of the inner work that opens us to the higher orders of self.

This work can have powerful effects on the healee as well as on the healer or therapist. It is critically important, therefore, that the therapist takes particular care that he or she uses these energies in a constructive manner that is in the best interests of the healee. The therapist must not fall into the maws of any of the four terrible dragons of self-delusion who are the enemies of Therapeutic Touch: fantasy, exaggeration, impulse, or wishful thinking, for they will also act to color the vital energies you are projecting to the healee.

Conscientiously pursued, this inner work can lead to a highly valued conscious personal knowing as you go within during the Therapeutic Touch interaction and explore the deeper levels of self. Tracing back or following the flow of your own consciousness in a self-search that is securely nested in a matrix of equilibrium, the work evolves into an act of interiority, an act of mindfulness that can help you acquire a dependable source of empowerment far beyond the most fanciful of fantasies.

However, you bring all of yourself to that moment, and how does the responsible therapist recognize what that "all" entails? Because it is the nature of the healing interaction for the healer to project a sense of vigor, selected feeling tones, outright emotions, and thoughts and aspirations to the healee, it is important to consider just what these congeries of personal stuff are that we sometimes unintentionally launch at the healee, along with our strong desire to help.

Perhaps the most potent emotions derive from our motivation to heal in the first place. These cohesive patterns of vital energies have functional attributes that we, in fact, call patterns—behavioral patterns such as habits, emotional dispositions, or moods. The last, mood, is a state we have all experienced, but it is also one that is the most vaguely defined. Our ignorance about this most powerful ally, mood, is unfortunate. Through recent bioscientific findings, this homely, commonplace feeling state has been shown to be central to stimulating essential neuropeptides throughout the body, such as the endorphins and enkephalins that control levels of pain and stimulate the body's immunosystem into action. Therefore, as persons committed to helping others, we need to be most keenly aware of this largely unspecified but common disposition. Exploration of the Self 10. "Natural Touchstones of Emotional States," below, was designed to assist in the fundamental recognition of this feeling state.

EXPLORATIONS OF THE SELF 10

Natural Touchstones of Emotional States

Note: Perhaps the most direct way of apprehending our own moods is at the physical level, where there are several natural basic touchstones or criteria that may sharpen our perception of a feeling state at a particular time. You can be either standing or sitting to do the exercise below; however, standing will put you in a more aware position to capture clues to your mood.

Materials

Journal, or writing pad, and pen.

Procedure

1. Begin by centering your consciousness.

2. Feel the pull of gravity on your extremities and note whether you are strongly resisting its pull, are restless under its constant pressure, or are simply unaware of gravity's effect on you.

3. Now become aware of your balance as you stand or sit. Do you feel as though your torso is tilting to one side? Are you leaning forward or backward? Do you feel tension in your neck? Your lower back? How would you describe your physical state?

4. Turn your attention to your breathing and become aware of its pattern of inhalation and exhalation. Where is your breathing occurring? Mostly high in your chest? Does it feel as though the inhalation of your breath reaches down to your abdomen? Do you feel that you are holding your breath, or do you feel well ventilated? Is there a feeling tone associated with how you are using your breath?

5. Now turn your attention to how the light in the room is affecting you. Is there tension in the muscles around your eyes? Brief, rapid movements of the eye are natural; however, is there anything unusual or annoying in these saccadic eye movements? How do your eyes feel when you close them for a moment or two? Do you feel relaxed with your eyes closed, or can you hardly wait to open them again?

6. Are you aware of sounds in the area about you? What is the nature of these sounds? How are they affecting you?

7. Take a few slow, deep breaths, and consider what these physical signs are telling you about your mood. Jot down notes on the impressions your physical senses invoke in you.

8. Scan the list when you are done. Be alert to any associated ideas or feelings that well up within you, and as you do so note them in the margin of your journal.

9. Reread all of your notes, including the associated ideas, and note the feeling state or mood that arises. The critical question to come to grips with, of course, is: Would you want that pattern of vital energies to be included in projections you might direct to a healee during a Therapeutic Touch session? It requires a straight answer that only you can supply, and it is important that you do so.

Projecting Emotions During Therapeutic Touch

Few in our culture are aware of the background swirl of personal, free-wheeling feelings and desires as we go through the routine of daily activities. As Therapeutic Touch therapists, it is well to remember what we are doing, or not doing, as we project our own vital energies supposedly in the service of others. Simply said, when the healer is upset, he or she also radiates that disturbance. To shift a possibly indifferent emotional posture into a conscious, responsible voice, review your responses to Exploration of the Self 10, and consider how you might develop this exercise into a personal homework task for healees in your Therapeutic Touch practice for whom it might be appropriate. This exercise is simple, encourages objectivity, and might be helpful to you both, for there is no better way to learn than to teach another.

The way we use inchoate emotions as unformed, or underformed, tatterings of vital-energy flow can be crucial to our health. For instance, after unresolved or unrecognized anger a person often feels helpless, depleted of energy, and may show signs of physical or emotional exhaustion. Or, a person who has unconsciously submitted to depression may appear to be in a state of deep lethargy, unaware of life about him or her, and frequently loses interest in primal needs, eating inadequately and drinking insufficient amounts of fluids. Similarly, unacknowledged fear immobilizes, unrealized resentment slowly erodes our vital-energy level, unresolved guilt stifles spontaneity and creativity, and overwhelming grief often disconnects us from those who care. These amorphous, poorly patterned emotional states, nevertheless, can importantly affect the autonomic nervous system and the endocrine system, to name but two major sites that can readily detract from a state of well-being. If provoked in sufficient degree, the ante goes up, and so vital organs, such as the heart, the digestive system, or the brain might also become affected. The story of secondary sequelae can go on and on, and so it is important preventive work to help those who do not know how to break through patterns of automatic and unconscious reactions, and replace them with conscious inner work.

Pattern Recognition of Human Energies

Pattern recognition of what we perceive is one of the fundamental ways by which we understand the world about us. The pattern acts as a model or example of the ideas associated with the confirmation and, as the pattern is analyzed, we get an understanding of its attributes.

Where we find pattern recognition most useful in Therapeutic Touch is in the assessment phase. In this, we use all the senses at our disposal, so that when we first see the healee we do an "eyeball" evaluation of his or her condition, in effect asking: What does it look like? That initial inquiry sparks a subjective appraisal that cuts to our gut reactions for confirmation, and we question again: What does it feel like? Most frequently in our culture there is a quick, rational check that evokes a more relational evaluation as we consider: What is the connection between the interacting factors? With adequate breadth of mind, a further, more united assessment might occur to us as we consider the context of this relationship in the greater scheme of things—for instance, from the perspective of the greater good. However, from the purview of Therapeutic Touch these simple data are not enough. Therapeutic Touch seeks indications of the healee's condition beyond the obvious physical, the provoked psychological, the tightly articulated intellectual, or the categorized philosophical states. The Therapeutic Touch assessment seeks out the underlying dynamic bases of these conditioned states in the vital-energy field itself. The kinds of information we look for have to do with a sense of the symmetry of the vital-energy field and its reciprocal factors, homeodynamic flow and fundamental integrity.

The Therapeutic Touch therapist must go beyond the simple components of logic, for the critical effects of the vital-energy field deal with the nonphysical in a dynamic way where laws of being have a strangeness of their own that requires a different type of intelligence, a knowing that extends beyond the five major senses.

This searching beyond our usual sensorium for information on the healee's condition increases and deepens our sensitivity to others. However, this process requires an empathy that, if poorly handled, can slide into a too-close identification with the client. So there is another caution to consider: Instead of the therapist helping the healee with the problem, the therapist him- or herself becomes the problem. Therefore, it is important to self-monitor your own motivation to insure an honest ackowledgment of whose needs are being met by this relationship. However, if we are truly on-center, there is a fail-safe proviso in place; the centering process itself acts as an inner gauge of all that is not in balance, and so the question does not often arise. Nevertheless, it is the responsibility of the therapist to be self-aware. Therefore, more so than others, we each must be willing to be accountable for the wanderings of our own mind, the most important tool of our trade.

Sensitivity to Cues in the Vital-Energy Field

As noted in the previous chapter, the hand chakras are important centers of psychic awareness, and, therefore, under appropriate conditions, the cues perceived may constellate into a clear visualization of the healee's condition. Such intelligence is as precious as it is rare, for it permits the possibility of using the Therapeutic Touch assessment as a basis for a new way of communication with others of similar mindfulness.

In the Therapeutic Touch assessment, we translate the direct experience of the healee's vital-energy field in terms of cues. Cues are sensed irregularities or "differences" that indicate to the therapist various kinds of imbalances in the field. They are patterns of vital-energy flow. In fact, everything in the universe is a distinctive pattern of energy flow. Nature talks to us in patterns, and through pattern recognition, we get a hint of the meaning of an object's organization.

With practice, we can be sensitive not only to spatial cues but also to rhythmic cues that act as a background to the interactions of the vital-energy field. This should not be surprising for, as discussed previously, prana is said to derive from the element Vayu, whose innate characteristic is rhythm. This signature is imprinted on the vital systems of the body through which prana streams. When something goes awry, it is most disconcerting to pick up cues that are dyssynchronous. As a nurse, one of my most awesome experiences has been finding significant rhythmic changes in cues in the vital-energy fields of patients who have had mechanical organ replacements—such as cardiac pacemakers—or who are connected to high-tech machinery that simulates vital functions—such as a kidney dialysis machine, a lung respirator, or an intravenous lock. Often the natural rhythmic background of the healee's vital-energy field is replaced by a perceptible mechanistic beat that resembles the periodic oscillations of the embodied machine-works. In the case of the kidney dialysis machine that has been used for a long period of time, I have noticed that the mimicked machine-like cadence will persist in the energy field, even when the person is not attached to the machine. Although these effects have been clinically verified by many other Therapeutic Touch therapists who have worked with me, this is only one of many findings in clinical Therapeutic Touch practice that calls for further rigorous, controlled study and broad theoretical consideration of the confirmed effects before we can adequately evaluate what this change in fundamental life-rhythm signifies.

Additionally, cues in the vital-energy fields of other than human beings can be assessed in the same way as we do healees' fields and, in fact, this can become the focus for interesting and challenging games, as will be presented in chapter 8. For instance, we can quite readily pick up cues in the vital-energy fields of seeds. Seeds have a strongly vital life core—and, therefore, 90-foot oaks from little acorns do grow. I found out about this striking high-potency feature several years ago when I was adopted by a Native American family and given a medicine bag with several items in it that I was taught to use. Two items particularly interested me—corn and hoddentin—which is the pollen of the mature cattail plant. Although they are both essentially seeds, each is used in a different way, and I wondered whether their life energies were qualitatively different. I did a Therapeutic Touch assessment on each of them and it intrigued me to find that they were, in fact, different. This study was so much fun that I made up a game, which I recount in Explorations of the Self 11. "Seed Ideas," so that you can enjoy it, too. Two or more people can play this game, or a single person can explore its possibilities.

EXPLORATIONS OF THE SELF 11

Seed Ideas

Materials

1. A small handful each of unadulterated corn kernels or corn meal, hoddentin (pollen of cattails), and small pebbles about the same size as the corn kernels.

2. Three small cloth bags made of the same material. Into each bag put one small handful of one of the three items noted above.

3. Scorecard and pen.

Procedure

1. All participants begin by centering.

2. In the case of 2 persons playing this game, a toss of a coin decides who will be first; we will call that person, "A."

3. "A" stands in front of a table and closes his or her eyes or is blindfolded.

4. The other person, "B," places the three bags on the table directly in front of "A" in any order; however, the bags should be separated from each other by about 6 inches. When the bags are in place, "B" lets "A" know and stands aside.

5. Blindfolded, "A" can approach the table as closely as he or she wishes. When "A" is in place, the hands are outstretched, and a Therapeutic Touch assessment is done of each bag without touching them, or, one at a time, "A" can place a bag on the palm of one hand and do the assessment with the other hand held above the bag. "A" describes the field overlying each bag, and states what he or she thinks each bag contains.

6. The contents of each bag are verified. Two points are awarded for each bag correctly identified. If "A" identifies all three bags, a special prize of 10 points are awarded.

7. "B" is now blindfolded, "A" arranges the three bags on the table, all take a moment to center, and then "B" tries to determine the contents of the three bags, as above.

8. Each person can have three tries. The person or team with the highest score wins.

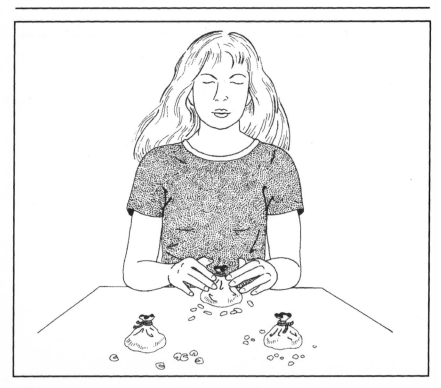

FIGURE 8: Assessing energy of "mystery" bags

Note: The qualities that I found in the vital-energy fields of the corn and the hoddentin were distinctly different. The corn had a pronounced, penetrating, and focused heat. The heat was clearly defined, surprisingly intense, and unvaryingly steady. The hoddentin was a finer, but nevertheless robust energy, which felt cool but not cold. There seemed to be an even rhythm to it and a generalized quality throughout the field that may be best described as "electric glow." The characteristic quality of the pebbles seemed to depend on their source. The most fun I had was when I substituted little quartz crystals for the pebbles. If I'm feeling adventurous and have somebody to play with, we separate out the different kinds of seeds from about a pound of bird seeds, so that we have a handful each of sunflower seeds, millet, and niger seeds, for example. We cover each small pile and then, as in the "Seed Ideas" exploration, above, we try to determine the characteristics of their life energies.

This game serves to exercise our hand chakras in an interesting way, and my friends and I have fun doing it. Sometimes we sprout the seeds to see what kind of difference that may make in our perceptions. It's a great way to spend a stormy day indoors, perk up the cabin-fever days of January and February, or transform a day of simple, garden-variety blahs. So, enjoy!

The Validity of Touch Without Contact

As noted in the exercise above, the Therapeutic Touch assessment is described as the use of the hand chakras, after the centering of the self, by utilizing the palms of the hands several inches away from the healee's body surface as sensors to locate cues that indicate imbalances in the vital-energy field. That may be a limited exercise because, under certain conditions, the therapist might want to place the hands directly on the healee's body or, with practice, learn how to use other chakras in the Therapeutic Touch assessment.

Picking up information by touching an object has never been questioned in Western society, because most of the anatomical sites corresponding to touch have been located and their physical effects have been measured. For instance, it is accepted that the largest part of the sensory strip of the cerebral cortex is concerned with touch and, therefore, we can pick up more physical data through the use of touch than by any other sense organ. We know that touch can cause considerable physiological effects because studies have demonstrated that touch results in the occurrence of chemical changes in the brain. Touch also effects a significant change in breathing patterns, and lowers the pulse rate and blood pressure. In addition, touch acts to calm people who are upset, and helps the individual to deal with stress in a manner that is quantifiable.

The "touch" that is central to Therapeutic Touch—in which the hands may either rest upon the healee's body tissues to gain information or be used as sensors several inches from the body, as the situation calls for—cannot use such measurement-based criteria for its nonphysical aspects. The too-simple reason for this is that instruments to reliably measure the dynamic space that is the matrix for vital energies have not been invented yet, and such tools are the recognized basic validators of empirical research. (Of course, in the West we have not always remembered that "our" mathematics draws upon other cultures' ideas. For example, the foundational concept of zero—without which there would be no reliable "measure"—was developed by the ancient Arabs. The ability to correctly design calendars by which the Maya predicted future astronomical events with scientific surety also gives us pause.)

However, ancient teaching, this time of India, helps us find validation for the practice of touching therapeutically without the therapist contacting the healee's skin, as often occurs in Therapeutic Touch. Once again, reference to the Upanishads finds the foundational ideas that underlie this concept so central to Therapeutic Touch. The basic assumption upon which validation rests is that we, as individuals, receive information of all sensory data through physiological portals, gateways or thresholds, which we in the West call "sensory organs." However, the crucial point at which the dominant contemporary view departs from the ancient is that the Upanishads state that the sensory organs are only the physical instruments by which the data are retrieved. The mind, by focusing its faculties, exerting its attention, and synthesizing the incoming data and consequent reaction to it, together with its relation to intuition (*buddhi*) and its identification with self, works through the sense organs and actually empowers them (Avalon, pp. 59-64). In this sense, we could say that the physical "paraphernalia" acts much like a robotic probe. Since the essential power is derived from the mind, the literature states that one who is learned in the process may accomplish, by mind, all the functions of the sense organs—that is, without touch, without use of the sense organs themselves. Within this context, the Therapeutic Touch assessment (which was conceived as, and continues to be, a modality that usually does not use the hand per se, but does use the hand chakras to contact the body and its vital energies) receives its validity from the heedful attention and conscious expression of the centered mind, a different-than-usual source of intelligence. From this perspective we can acknowledge that touch, particularly as it is used in Therapeutic Touch, is a "telereceptor" acting at a distance, as are the other four major physical senses: hearing, which acts through vibratory stimuli; seeing, which functions through the photons of electromagnetic radiation; and taste and smell, which operate through chemical molecules.

The Effects of Therapeutic Touch on the Therapist

The knowledgeable Therapeutic Touch therapist recognizes that the understanding of the therapeutic use of the vital-energy field is a major, but not the only, indication of expertise. Of equal, if not greater importance is how knowledge can be applied to a person's life. The consistent practice of centering sharpens the recognition of the subtle world within, and clarifies the realization that its functions are within conscious reach. As the therapist hones the fine skills of intentionality in life, the Therapeutic Touch practices become more focused, coherent, and in alignment with the goals set for each Therapeutic Touch engagement. The therapist also learns to accept the powers of compassion as ally and to allow them to work their grace in their own time and in their own way during the healing enactment. These perceptions act to foster a high level of confidence (another ally) in the helping and healing of those in need.

There is a synergistic effect on the therapist who has a committed lifestyle of centering the personal consciousness to understand the more subtle energies that affect human beings, and to consciously sensitize his or her linkages with the higher orders of self. Responding to the needs of the healee with compassion, the Therapeutic Touch therapist works mainly through the heart chakra, which, as noted in chapter 3, has a natural affinity to the sense of touch. These interacting features foster in the therapist a sense of oneness with all of Nature, and the associated upwelling sense of aspiration and identification serves to awaken the intuitive capacity and to further sensitize us to the promptings of the inner self. Concomitantly, the compelling power of this united outreach breaks through the more restricted patterns of conditioned and habituated vital-energy flows. Over time, the consequent repatterning sets up nodes of opportunity for the establishment of new relationships within the vital-energy field. These new relationships are but an indication of a creative set that can be imprinted upon the unencumbered pattern of the being of the therapist. In health, that person is self-organizing, continually unfolding the potentials of his or her implicate being, and constantly changing—and, therefore, naturally primed to make therapeutic use of a creative act. In the healing matrix, we are faced with the realization that not only can these become our own characteristics, but also that the opportunity is there for the healee. Within this frame, as the Therapeutic Touch therapist learns to recognize his or her own potentialities, there is an increased appreciation of the potentials of others.

The Different Universes of Healer and Healee

Contrary to the therapist—who would be very foolish if he or she did not have a belief system that was in consonance with what he or she was doing—the healee does not need to have faith in the Therapeutic Touch process for it to succeed. However, over time, we have noted that it is important that the healee has an open mind, and is willing to relax and accept the therapist's help. Given these very few prerequisites, Therapeutic Touch can bring into functional compatibility many critical basic body processes, such as respiration, metabolism, blood circulation, nerve impulses, biochemical exchange, and acid-base balance. For the healee undergoing Therapeutic Touch, the most frequent statement after the session is that a deep sense of peace is felt. This is described as a feeling of being slightly removed from the hubbub of daily life, and having a decided sense of the interplay of fine energies throughout the body or just a bit beyond it, in the vital-energy field. It will quite often also be verbalized that ". . . other-than-ordinary aspects of myself come into play," and the healee now feels differently about him- or herself and about persons with whom he or she interacts. Clinically, respirations are now fuller and deeper; the musculature feels less tense, more relaxed; the healee feels calmer and more in control; there is less or no pain, and a greater sense of well-being.

Given these positive features of Therapeutic Touch, it is not unusual for the novice therapist or the casual observer to identify with the healee in an assumption that both healee and healer are having similar experiences. This is not actually so, and needs to be examined. Besides the fact that their motivations differ—the healee is motivated by a desire to be well or no longer in pain, whereas the therapist's motivation arises out of compassion for the healee and a desire to help or heal—the consequences of the Therapeutic Touch interaction are fundamentally different for each.

The effect on each is profound; however, for the healer this is dominated by a sense of purposefulness that arises out of a command of the forces of intentionality, whereas the effect on the healee is a sense of peacefulness and well-being. Studies have shown that the state of consciousness has changed for each of them, but the Therapeutic Touch therapist's electroencephalographic tracing of brain waves demonstrates that during the Therapeutic Touch session there is a finely synchronous, high beta state, which indicates a keenly alert, coordinated state of awareness in both cerebral hemispheres. The healee's electroencephalographic readings indicate an alpha state of relaxation, even though the eyes are open (Krieger, Peper, and Ancoli, 1979). In addition, both healer and healee have a firm sense of confidence in the process, but the object of that confidence is different. The confidence of the therapist is in the integral dynamics of the Therapeutic Touch process; the healee's source of confidence is in the competent actions of the therapist. At the end of the session, there is an acknowledged bonding between the therapist and the healee. For the therapist, this bonding arises as an aspect of the transpersonal experience in which he or she has consciously engaged during the Therapeutic Touch interaction; for the healee, this close relationship may arise out of admiration for the therapist or it may blossom during the session as an unconscious urge when ". . . other-than-usual aspects of myself come into play." Graphically stated, differences between therapist and healee may look like table 1, below.

Who are the people we are trying to help or to heal? In the typical "sick" pattern of behavior, the person appears to withdraw to an unusual extent to some inner place of self-consciousness, to be cut off from the daily activities of living or to be set apart from the natural constant and potent interaction between the universe and the individual that most of us take for granted and consider to be our linkage to "the whole" of life and living. The healee feels outside the loop and has lost control. On the contrary, when you have a sense of well-being, you feel that you are in synch with the universe. Under this impetus life is more or less easy, there seems to be a rhythm to living as you go with the flow, and the events in that flow seem to have a certain predictability. This is not so for the healee whom the flow may have taken on a tortuous and unpredictable route, and each step on that path can provoke a disquieting anxiety, an intense pain, or a gut-wrenching fear. Nevertheless, those with some experience with Therapeutic Touch, to whom centering is an intrinsic part of their lifestyle, will agree with Dora Kunz's findings that the Therapeutic Touch therapist can learn to mentally reach out from his or her moorings in the innermost self to the inner self of the healee with such clarity that, in the felt impact of that intentionality, the healee can acknowledge that he or she, too, is rooted in that timeless realm of equilibrium and serenity. The healee will realize that he or she is not alone and, as Kunz puts it so well, ". . . he [or she] will find the ability to endure."

TABLE 1
The Different Universes of Therapist and Healee

A. THERAPEUTIC TOUCH THERAPIST	B. HEALEE
Nurtured by:	*Nurtured by:*
compassion	mood, which stimulates
centered state of consciousness	neuropeptides
knowledgeable intentionality	relaxation response,
	facilitates immunosystem
Activated by:	*Activated by:*
skills of: direction	resonant wave of
modulation	endocrine change that
unruffling	also activates the
	immunosystem
Rooted in:	*Rooted in:*
orientation toward higher	will to change (out of
orders of self	which the lesson of illness
	is learned)

The Reality of the Transpersonal

This glimpse of the farther reaches of the Therapeutic Touch interaction has profound implications. It suggests that there is more to the process than a worldview in which streams of energy interpenetrate the biosphere and are cycled in biorhythms that flow on biochemical tides patterned by field forces that are vitalized by prana. We begin to see that this biophysical scenario is too generalized, not necessarily human, and conceptually sterile unless we also posit an organizational base that hearkens to a different kind of intelligence and conscious mind. Then we perceive that a valid role for Therapeutic Touch could be the provision of a life-affirmative set through which the mind can be more fully realized in its urge to fulfill its innate directive toward self-awareness.

Here we pause, because our culture does not readily recognize the suprarational and the unmeasurable. However, if conceptual frames of other cultures are admitted to this discussion, we might see beyond our bias. The ancient Chinese, for instance, remembered that we were integral with the universe and, in the context of that whole, the enemy was not Nature, but our insensitivity to her forces working through us. From such a perspective, we could affirm the possibility of a continuing inner evolution that proceeds beyond the largely instinctive biopsychological growth and development to an unfolding of new consciousness that is fostered by the humane urge to help or to heal others.

It is the act of centering in the context of compassionately helping/healing others that opens us to the finer impulses of the inner self where new ideas, new actions, new strivings, and new aspirations can thrive. The act of centering forces coherence out of the usual stream of imaged representations that flow by as casual notions, metaphors, information, and memories, and imprints on them a clearly patterned structure oriented toward meeting the needs of the healee. By virtue of the primacy of centering, Therapeutic Touch can become a transpersonal act as the therapist allows the inner life to vitally interact with the outer life and thereby to thoroughly imbue that social overlay with a spark of its own essence. This intimate relationship can then bring into its sphere of influence a unique energetic, the finer forces of the higher orders of self. We can observe the enactment of this transpersonal dynamic during times of true—that is, unobstructed—acts of compassion.

The concept of transpersonal dimensions to consciousness arose out of Maslow's studies of peak experiences of exceptional people (Maslow, 1968). In particular, he recognized the reality of experiences of the higher orders of self in our lives. The prefix "trans" indicates states of consciousness in the individual that go beyond those we usually are aware of in everyday life. The term "transpersonal consciousness" implies that consciousness may not always be restricted to the physical body and the brain. Tart more fully defined the transpersonal by calling further attention to the implication that there may be other kinds of consciousnesses with which we can interact than those we usually employ (Tart, 1975).

There are several levels of transpersonal experiences that are considered potential in human beings, and they are said to originate in the deep unconscious. As noted previously, Therapeutic Touch provides a climate in which the transpersonal has an opportunity to arise. It is, therefore, quite important to thoughtfully consider Wilbur's statement in reference to the transpersonal: that what one goes beyond is the personal ego, and his caution that the individual must develop a healthy and stable ego before he or she can successfully transcend that ego. He adds, ". . . failure to do so can result in a pathological state often accompanied by high psychological stress" (Wilbur, 1980).

These comments should be considered seriously by all who contemplate making the practice of Therapeutic Touch a lifeway. Euphoria is not what we are after. The personal challenge is to design the conditions of our life in such fashion that this universal force can flow through without our individual inadequacies hindering or warping its passage. Without a doubt, it is a challenge. Expertly done, however, this is a fine way to become a human support system for those in need and an excellent goal for those who wonder, *"Why do I want to be healer?"*

DYNAMIC FEATURES OF THE THERAPEUTIC TOUCH PROCESS

Allies of Healing

"They died so often," she said. Otelia, a medical doctor and old friend, was sitting with me at the side of a lively rippling stream one summer afternoon as we discussed Therapeutic Touch. She had strongly supported Therapeutic Touch since Dora Kunz and I began to develop it in 1972, and whenever we saw each other she would ask me for an update on activities concerning it. I had just mentioned that paralytic ileus, a paralysis of the intestinal wall that very often occurred after any abdominal operation, was one of the conditions we routinely treated successfully with Therapeutic Touch. Otelia, who was then about ninety-four years old, was obviously startled by the casualness of my remarks. She was quite still for a full moment as she gazed at the rapidly moving waters, and then she told me that when she was a young intern, in the early part of the twentieth century, she and her colleagues dreaded being assigned to patients scheduled for abdominal operations, because of the high post-operative mortality rate when the seemingly inevitable paralytic ileus developed. "Even now," she quietly said, "hearing this about Therapeutic Touch, I feel as though a prayer has been answered."

It was my turn to be jolted. By that time, 1990, those of us in the health professions who worked with surgical patients had been using Therapeutic Touch successfully for ten years to treat paralytic ileus. It had proved to be a safe and useful intervention and we had lost our fear of the problem, so that I had all but forgotten that paralytic ileus once had been considered deadly.

(In an odd bit of real-time synchronicity, a short while after writing these paragraphs, I received a phone call from a friend who was a Therapeutic Touch therapist. Crystal was in the intensive-care unit of a large hospital in Toronto, Canada, and was calling to tell me of an unusual incident. She had given a Therapeutic Touch treatment to a near-comatose patient, thought to be terminally ill. A floor nurse had accompanied her to the bedside. She was noncommittal but curious as she watched the overhead monitor of the patient's vital signs as Crystal worked with the patient. Suddenly, about three minutes into the Therapeutic Touch session, the nurse let out a shriek that brought staff within hearing distance scrambling into the room. Pointing to the monitor, the nurse directed everyone's gaze to the readings, which were now unaccountably reversed to normal and had stabilized. In a comedic turn of events, the patient, an elderly woman, opened her eyes, smiled, and said, pointing to her body, "Would you please scratch me, just about there?" and then promptly fell into a normal, sound sleep. The staff was startled by the events and offered comments such as, "Sensational!" "Unbelievable!" and "If I hadn't seen it with my own eyes...." I said to Crystal, "That does sound remarkable. What had been the matter with the lady?" The answer: "Oh, paralytic ileus." Needless to say, even I was amazed at the synchronicity of writing in New York about the success of treating paralytic ileus with Therapeutic Touch at the same time that Crystal was exemplifying that success in Toronto, Canada. I think I can hear the lilt of Otelia's quiet laughter!)

Allies of Self-Healing

Over the years, I have found that the body system most sensitive to Therapeutic Touch is the autonomic nervous system (ANS) and, consequently, Therapeutic Touch could be used successfully with a large number of ANS dysfunctions. The next most sensitive to

Therapeutic Touch were dysfunctions of the lymphatic system, the circulatory system, and the genitourinary system, with problems of the musculoskeletal system following closely behind. However, the concept of body-system sensitivity did not work fully; for instance, only certain dysfunctions of the endocrine system were helped by Therapeutic Touch while others were not (Krieger, 1993). Although at the time of this writing, twenty-seven doctoral dissertations have been completed and accepted, and eighteen postdoctoral researches have been reported, valid reasons for sensitivity or nonsensitivity to Therapeutic Touch still elude us.

The healthy physical body itself is marvelously resistant to disease; its makeup includes a staggering number of redundancies and, therefore, it can tolerate a great deal of assault. More than a half-century ago, Canon, who conceived the idea that the body maintains a physiological homeostasis, noted that the physical body could function in times of stress even if:

- two-thirds of each kidney was removed

- nine-tenths of adrenal tissue was excised

- only one-fifth of the thyroid gland functioned adequately

- only one-fifth of the pancreas was producing insulin

- only one-fourth of the liver was intact and functioning.

He also remarked that about ten feet of the normal twenty-three feet of the small intestine could be removed and the body would still maintain its integrity, and that very little of the large intestine was of critical importance. In addition, he pointed out that blood sugar and calcium levels in the blood, systolic blood pressure, lung capacity, and large areas of the brain were all greater than they need be for homeostasis to be maintained (Canon, 1932).

From this data we realize that humans have evolved in a privileged fail-safe mode. It would seem, then, that the healing effort need only be slight in order to tilt a person toward wellness. And there is a veritable plethora of built-in allies that protect the body and heal it:

- A first line of protection and healing is the response of the immune system. The infallible ability of this system to recognize objects foreign to the body and regard them as invaders to be attacked is remarkable. Because of this reliable ability to recognize features outside of itself and respond appropriately for survival, the immune system now is regarded as a type of second brain.

- When exposed to trauma, shock, or stress, the autonomic nervous system will instantaneously react to protect the body. Most of these reactions compose or bolster the survival instinct, which most frequently acts at the unconscious level.

- The thyroid gland is another confederate in this alliance to maintain the body in a state of well-being. A central function of the thyroid gland is the anabolic-catabolic process of building up and breaking down cellular structures, a process that reinforces wound healing.

- A set of endocrine glands that does yeoman services for the body's welfare is the adrenals. These two small, but highly potent, glands are situated over the kidneys as small caps, and are essential to life itself. The adrenals are very sensitive to Therapeutic Touch, and easily and safely accessed (Krieger, 1993).

- There are several structures in the brain of importance to healing and maintaining a state of well-being; however, of signal importance are the thalamic bodies, one in each hemisphere of the brain. They serve as relay stations for incoming sensory data. In this process they filter out inappropriate or overloading stimuli that, unchecked, would overwhelm the body's physiological homeodynamics.

- A deeper brain structure, the limbic system, filters out overloads of emotional stimuli. This system enables the withdrawal of conscious awareness from intolerable or sick situations, and thereby acts as access to sanctuary during trying times.

- In addition to these natural features of the body, other notable allies are body tissues that normally display a high capacity for regeneration, such as are found in bone, the liver, the skin, and the peripheral nerves; they can be counted upon to heal quickly under normal circumstances.

Therapeutic Touch as a Growth Experience in Personal Knowledge

What do we know that helps us to utilize these natural allies and, when necessary, to go beyond them with Therapeutic Touch skills? Dora Kunz and I have spent almost a quarter-century probing this question and seeking out the theoretical bases to which Therapeutic Touch adheres. A brief resumé of individual and combined contributions would include:

- A Human Vital-Energy Field Model (Kunz)

- Model of Therapeutic Touch as a Human Potential (Krieger)

- Conceptual Framework of Compassion and Order in the Universe (Kunz)

- Conceptual Framework of Intentionality and Compassion as Empowerment Bases of Therapeutic Touch (Krieger)

- Conceptual Framework of Conscious Centeredness as the Critical Variables in Therapeutic Touch (Kunz and Krieger)

- The Therapeutic Touch Assessment as an Analogic Retrieval System (Krieger)

- Model of Therapist's Deep-Role Identity During Therapeutic Touch Assessment, and Counter-Role Identity During the Rebalancing Process (Krieger)

- Conceptual Frame of Birth-Life-Death Continuum as Natural Universal Law (Kunz):

1. All components of the universe are engaged in a continuous cycling through the processes of birth, life, and death.

2. Therefore, change is an apparent universal constant.

3. Consequently, the therapist should not feel personally responsible for either the successes or the failures of Therapeutic Touch.

In addition, there are several reliable principles underlying Therapeutic Touch practice:

- You don't stop at your skin; that is, the individual as a localized vital-energy field extends beyond the physical and biological limitations of the skin.

- During the Therapeutic Touch assessment, the therapist apprehends vitality, emotions, and thought as human energies in the healee's vital-energy field.

- Balancing the human vital-energy field is analogous to a general principle of opposites.

- The skills of Therapeutic Touch are predicated upon a sense of compassion and order in the universe, and are empowered by a background of centered consciousness in the therapist.

- Attention (mind) directs and modulates the vital-energy field.

- Less is more; that is, the greater the trauma, the gentler should Therapeutic Touch be done, and for shorter periods of time.

- Chakras are centers of different kinds of consciousness that are intrinsic to both the humanness and the uniqueness of each individual.

- There is an interesting and valid analogy between DNA and the chakras, in that neither of them can be structurally altered, except by the individual him- or herself. However, through Therapeutic Touch, the vital-energy flows that are transformed by the chakras as they enter the domain of the personal self can be modulated and modified in the interest of the well-being of the healee.

• Lastly, and unalterably—when in doubt, don't do anything. Refer the healee to someone more knowledgeable.

The vital-energy field is the major domain of expertise in Therapeutic Touch practice. The therapist gets to know and appreciate the nature of the vital-energy field by perceiving cues with the hand chakras. This interaction then indicates to him or her whether the field is in a state of balance or imbalance. The primary characteristics of the well-integrated field as perceived by the therapist are: flow, rhythm, pattern, balance, and symmetry, and indications of a background implicate order. Major cues that indicate a state of imbalance in the vital-energy field are: a sense of congestion or undue pressure in the vital-energy flow; irregular or uncoordinated and discordant motion or vibration in the field; a lack of symmetry in the arrangement of features in the field; or a significant deviation in the perceived temperature of the field.

These characteristics are imprinted on the prana streaming in the vital-energy field. As noted in chapter 3, there are five subsystems of the universal life force, or prana, that are assimilable at this time. Of these subsystems, I would think from their descriptions that the one called "vyana" is probably the system most accessible to Therapeutic Touch. Vyana gains access to the individual through the splenic chakra, and then it permeates and streams through the whole body, vivifying it, and making possible muscular movement, blood circulation, metabolic function, and the distribution of vitality itself. If this hunch is true, it would be a major clue to the broad therapeutic reach of the Therapeutic Touch process.

Modifiers of Vital Energy

It is not always clear that only one aspect of Therapeutic Touch is the offering to help or to heal; apparently there is a wide spectrum in the ability to use prana. When doing the Therapeutic Touch assessment with people who are very ill, the therapist is trying very hard to ascertain how to help the healee and, therefore, is open to the full brunt of the healee's vital-energy field. At this time, the therapist may be quite vulnerable to the needs of the healee. The healee's depletion of energy can be readily noticeable as subtle but felt movement, for overflow of prana from the healthy therapist to the needy healee is rapid and direct. However, this conferral can also go unnoticed, not only during Therapeutic Touch, but also during the daily activities of laypersons and therapists, when they are in proximity to a greatly debilitated person. The flow of prana from stronger to weaker localized vital-energy fields seems to be a natural, universal, covert occurrence when two or more people gather. Under excessive conditions, the ill person has been termed a "sapper" of vital energy or, if the condition is chronic and extreme, the term "slurper" has been applied. This is not cause for undue alarm for, in either case, the aware therapist is in control of his or her intentionality and will act to maintain a healthy climate for both the healee and healer.

Soberly considered, it has to be acknowledged that the usual therapeutic exchange acts itself out in a mutually satisfying way, for the healing act does have a positive side. There are those who could be called "up-lifters," who freely project energy for the well-being of others—for instance, those who have the charisma to inspire others. And there are "stimulators," who are able to ignite the imagination of others for altruistic purposes or for high enthusiasm for a project or a cause, such as the cause for self-healing.

All these modifiers of human energy can be brought into the healing act; in fact, Nature herself can contribute positive modifiers of vital energy, and it needn't happen through human means. Historically, since the Egyptian dynasties, cats have been known to have a remarkably high level of prana and, therefore, have been venerated and protected in many cultures. Dogs and horses seem to have the ability to soothe and heal human emotional wounds. Scuba-diving with dolphins or swimming alongside a whale and gazing deeply into one of its eyes can arouse an overpowering sense of oneness with the universe. Electromagnetic sinks on the face of Earth, moving waters, high mountains—all have the ability to modify energies, and in all cultures they have been considered healing sites and sacred places.

Intentionality as Causal Factor

In Therapeutic Touch, the therapist helps the healee to find once again his or her own center. This rebalancing process involves a number of energy shifts or vital-energy repatternings. How this transfer of energy occurs has evaded scientific explanation. A possible analogy has been suggested: It is common knowledge in physics that it is the surrounding nonphysical field that carries the charge of electrons between objects, and this transfer occurs whether or not the objects come into contact. The explanation is that electrons in the outermost orbit at the molecular level are bound very loosely and, therefore, can be easily dislodged, carrying the electrical charge with them across the intervening space without a physical bridge to convey them. This happens whether the transport is between physical, inert objects or over a nerve synapse (which is also an "empty space") in the living body. The analogy is that something similar happens during Therapeutic Touch in the transfer of prana between the vital-energy fields of healer and healee.

In Therapeutic Touch, the impetus for this transport is the therapist's intentionality. As noted, intentionality is concerned with both the will to do and a conceptualization of a goal about how that might occur. In this sense, we might consider intentionality to be causal, rather than simply an "X" factor. However, that statement should not be accepted lightly; rather, as therapist you should know this as fact. Explorations of the Self 12. "The Personal Use of Intentionality," below, was designed to help you objectify your intentionality.

EXPLORATIONS OF THE SELF 12

The Personal Use of Intentionality

Note: Do this exploration when you can assure yourself of a half-hour of uninterrupted time with these questions. I suggest that you read these questions into a tape recorder, with a considerable pause between them to give you ample time to answer when the tape is played back. Be aware that there are alternate ways to do this exploration.

Materials

"Deep Dee" form, pen, and tape recorder.

Procedure

1. Place "Deep Dee" form and pen nearby, quietly center yourself, and either:

   • Go back in your memory to a recent time when you were engaged in a Therapeutic Touch interaction, and clearly visualize that scene. In particular, see yourself doing Therapeutic touch and try to identify with your state of consciousness at that time. Or,

   • Memorize the questions below, and answer them while you are actually doing Therapeutic Touch for a healee.

2. When you come to the rebalancing phase, objectify your sense of what you are doing and ask yourself the following questions while you continue to be engaged in the Therapeutic Touch process:

   • How do you perceive yourself using intentionality? For instance, do you have a preferred method for calling upon your intentionality? a particular frame of mind? a ritual?

   • What are you drawing upon within yourself as you use intentionality? For example, intuition? prayer? the higher orders of self?

- Do you align yourself with something during your act of intentionality? How would you describe it?

- Is there anything else that occurs at this time?

- How do you ascertain whether the objective of your intentionality was effectively attained?

3. When the rebalancing is done, make out the "Deep Dee" form and answer the questions.

4. After you have finished answering all the questions, read all your answers in one sitting. As you do so, additional thoughts may come to mind. Jot brief notes about these thoughts in the margin of the paper and come back to them later.

5. If you have done this Exploration with another person, discuss your experiences at this time, and compare them for similarities, differences, and new ideas about the process of intentionality.

6. Do you now have a fuller understanding of how you use intentionality? How would you defend the premise that your intentionality is/is not causal?

Intentionality can lead to significant change, if it is conscious, purposeful, and goal-oriented. In Therapeutic Touch these qualities assure that rebalancing will be a thoughtfully considered action; that is, it will be an act of mindfulness at work. This inner process can be objectively recorded, for instance, in studies using electroencephalography (Krieger, Peper, and Ancoli, 1979).

In Therapeutic Touch, intentionality becomes causal through the use of visualization, a process closely allied with creative imagination, which, itself, has nothing to do with fantasy. It appears to occur in three phases, as follows, or may be simultaneous with the Therapeutic Touch assessment of the healee:

1. The therapist sets up a field whose placement is determined during the assessment of the healee.

2. Intentionality wells up in the therapist in reference to decisions about the healing act.

3. Simultaneously, the therapist visualizes the route of the healing energies and guides them toward her or his goal.

The crucial point here is to make the visualization dynamically active. This activation seems to be facilitated by prompting a strong, positive emotion, such as love, compassion, or altruism. Once prompted, these feeling states seem to pour out spontaneously. The source appears to be a prior dedication to a person's highest ideal, whose signature vibratory response can come to awareness as either light or imagery, as its being vivifies the moment. If you can maintain your state of quiet centeredness and not waver from your committed intentionality, and at the same time be sensitive to the responses of your upper chakras, you can become aware of an unforgettable sense of the part being played in this healing moment, and its meaning for you becomes apparent. It is then that you realize that the opportunity to help or to heal is a rare privilege on the path to self-learning, or self-realization of the power of compassion.

This may be bliss, but it is also hard work to remain focused in your concentration on the process at hand in the service of the healee. And, of course, this is the name of the game. Most often the work of directing or modulating the vital-energy flows is done directly in the healee's energy field; that is, without making body contact, as may seem appropriate in the individual case. Or the therapist may wish to put one or both hands directly on the healee's body and use the chakra of the hand in body contact as an anchor or depositor of vital energy. In either case, the therapist uses the other hand chakra simultaneously to direct or modulate the flow, and to do this he or she clearly and strongly concentrates on the visualization of the vital- energy transfer. This ability is not dependent on the exertion of physical energy, but is an attribute of the field of the mind through the act of intentionality.

Intentionality Underlies Therapeutic Touch Skills

Therapeutic Touch is done gently, symmetrically, and, most important, rhythmically. Particular attention must be paid to maintaining this rhythmicity—for instance, doing it quickly does not necessarily imply that the act is also rhythmic. As noted several times, prana is an aspect of Vayu, whose major characteristic is rhythmicity. Today we would call Vayu a universal field (*tattva*, Skt.), much as the electromagnetic field is. In this context, prana could be thought of as an appropriate test object for that field, similar to the way iron filings are appropriate test objects for the electromagnetic field. Because prana is the test object of Vayu, it reflects the characteristic rhythmicity and, therefore, carrys forth that rhythmicity into the Therapeutic Touch process to make it "work" when we use the skills of directing or modulating.

Briefly stated, directing refers to regulating, guiding, or otherwise exercising a determining influence by directing the mind upon vital-energy flows in an intentional manner. Modulating vital energies refers to a wider variety of ploys: varying the intensity of the vital-energy flow; softening, dampening, or reducing the flow; or adjusting, shifting, or moderating the flow. Both "directing" and "modulating" can apply to either the use of vital energies flowing through the therapist, or to the way the therapist is attempting to support the healee's energy flows. The question of any difference is moot, for the Therapeutic Touch interaction of the therapist, as a human support system, and the healee is very complex at the healing moment and not easily describable, though the term "in resonance" might be valid and applicable.

Most frequently when the therapist is modulating energies he or she is applying intentionality to the redistribution of those energies, to tone up or to tone down the intensity of the energy state. The process is initiated upon inner command as directly and simply as we modulate the voice to convey emotional content. Visualizing the energy flow and suffusing that visualization with a color or colors seems to work best for most Therapeutic Touch therapists as they modulate the vital-energy flow. It is not the intention that the colors themselves make the change, but that visualizing colors helps the way the therapists think (see table 2). Similar effects can also occur through the use of sounds, or by engaging a mood or emotion.

TABLE 2
Colors Visualized During
Therapeutic Touch Modulation

VISUALIZED COLOR	PURPOSE	EXAMPLE
Royal blue	Calm, quiet sedate	Hypertensive states
Yellow gold	Stimulate, energize, quicken	Toxic conditions
Light green	Balance, energize	Extreme weakness
Clear light	Serenity, trust	Panic, fear
Rose	Gentle love	Emotional states, high anxiety, loneliness
Violet	Spiritual support	Crises, grief, dying

EXPLORATIONS OF THE SELF 13

Modulation as a Therapeutic Touch Skill

Note: This Exploration is designed for two people; one person will be the therapist and the other will be the healee. Through visualization, the therapist will be projecting color to the healee, instead of vital energy per se.

Materials

"Deep Dee" form, pen, blood pressure cuff and stethoscope (optional), and chair.

Procedure

1. Healee sits, therapist stands by his or her side

2. To begin the session, the therapist takes the pulse of the healee for one minute and, if appropriate apparatus is available, the blood pressure, and records these findings.

3. Both therapist and healee center.

4. The therapist does Therapeutic Touch assessment and briefly records the findings.

5. The therapist then centers again and modulates the healee's vital-energy field in a calming, quieting manner, using royal blue to "color" the energy being projected to the healee. Setting up a field over the healee's heart area, he or she saturates it with that sense of royal blue, that is, with a simulation of how that color (or "light") affects the body by, for instance, its vibrations or movement, or memories, emotions, or thoughts that the color evokes in the therapist.

6. After two to three minutes, as feels appropriate, the therapist sets up a field over the healee's internal carotids, on both sides of the neck, and again modulates with royal blue for two to three minutes.

7. The healee's pulse and blood pressure are taken again, and recorded.

8. If there is no significant lowering of the readings, the therapist repeats instructions 5 and 6, in reference to setting up a field over the healee's heart chakra and the internal carotids, and records the findings.

9. At this time the healee and the therapist should also record their subjective experiences.

10. Roles are now reversed and the steps are repeated.

11. After all recordings have been done, the "therapist" and the "healee" exchange experiences. What one new thing has been learned about how vital energies are modulated?

Unruffling as a Specific Act of Intentionality

Another way vital energies can be modulated is through the Therapeutic Touch technique known as "unruffling" (Krieger, 1993). Unruffling the healee's vital-energy field is essentially an act of specific intentionality. Therefore, underlying what may appear to be similar motions of the hands may, in fact, be subtle shades of difference in the intent of those gestures. In the world of nonphysical vital energies, it is the imprint of focused intent that effectively enforces subtle repatternings, more so by far than physical motions of pushing, pulling, or stuffing. Consequently, depending on the nuance of the intentionality behind the act, unruffling can serve several purposes during the overall Therapeutic Touch engagement.

The major function that unruffling can serve is to facilitate the vital-energy flows that are already in the healee's system. Unruffling can stimulate the vital-energy flow to pump in prana or, following an intentionality that is somewhat differently based, it can be used to reestablish the background rhythm of the vital-energy field as the therapist "evens out" and "smoothes" the energy flow. Used appropriately, this technique can be used to ameliorate symptoms of nausea and vomiting and the anxiety that often accompanies them, and to replace these symptoms with a refreshing relaxation response. Again, using only slight differences in gesture, unruffling twinned to intentionality can be used to break up very "sick" vital-energy patterns, such as the cues of congestion that indicate inwardly turned, static patterns of depression. With a variance in gesture coupled to a different intentionality, the cues of tense, poorly patterned buzzes and tinglings that indicate persistent, but inchoate, overactive flow in persons with abnormally high blood pressure, can be addressed. The very different responses in these last two examples speak clearly to the primacy of the intentionality that drives unruffling. How this happens is little understood at this time. (It does not take a large stretch of the imagination to wonder whether this humanized action at a distance might be clarified if we understood similar physical actions, such as the way a basketball or billard player uses intentionality expressed as "body English"—body movements intended to influence the course of a ball that is teetering in its path to, or around the edge of the basket or pocket—to actually "make" a ball fall into the basket or pocket, apparently in response to the player's body language.) Very often unruffling is done in conjunction with other types of modulation. As examples, unruffling used with a simultaneous modulation with royal blue can dramatically reduce elevated temperatures; used with slightly different gestures and coupled with a modulation of golden yellow, the unruffling during the Therapeutic Touch process will significantly hasten the healing of fractured bones from an average of six weeks to an average of two-and-a-half weeks. The various hand gestures are as much a direct reponse to the specific intentionality of the therapist as they are the sensitive reflectors of emotions and thought. Hand gestures are, therefore, gentle and soothing when intended to calm the vital-energy flows, forceful and vigorous when the purpose is to stimulate, or sweeping and wide-ranging when meant to rout out or break up patterns of vital-energy flow. Each motion mirrors the intentionality of the Therapeutic Touch therapist, with the movements of the hands and extremities punctuating the communication by specific gestures during the session.

Unruffling relaxes the healee as the therapist works to repattern bound energy flows and, as we have seen, the effect seems to assist the healee to absorb prana more efficiently as anxiety dissipates. As the healee receives and absorbs this continual flow, the symptoms fade and the healee's immune system defenses appear reinforced and strengthened.

Implications of the Relaxation Response

The most reliable clinical responses to Therapeutic Touch have been demonstrated to be due primarily to four factors:

- a profound and rapid relaxation response
- a significant reduction in pain

- an accelerated rate of healing
- the relief of psychosomatic symptoms

These consistent effects have given Therapeutic Touch entrée to a significant number of medical centers and health facilities around the world in the seventy-five countries where Therapeutic touch has been taught to date.

To separate out only one of these effects of Therapeutic Touch, the relaxation response in itself can have profound effects—it dilates the peripheral vascular system, dampens sympathetic nervous system reactions, and facilitates the response of the immune system. Because of these major effects, Therapeutic Touch therapists in emergency medical therapy, ambulance corps, search and rescue squads, ski patrols, firemen, and health personnel in intensive care, coronary care, and emergency trauma units use Therapeutic Touch for traumatized persons in shock or hysteria. It can be used during the pre-induction of anesthesia prior to high-risk surgery: during the prenatal care of the mother and throughout her labor and delivery of the newborn child; and before procedures that may be disquieting to patients, such as venipuncture and lumbar puncture. Therapeutic Touch also is frequently used to extend the analgesic and sedative effects of medications, reduce apprehension, promote restful sleep, and allay symptoms of autonomic nervous system dysfunctions. (See appendixes B and C for the current address of the Nurse Healers-Professional Associates, Inc., who have available updated lists of health facilities in both the United States and Canada where Therapeutic Touch is practiced and schools where it is taught.)

Effectiveness of Therapeutic Touch for Stress Regulation

The effectiveness of Therapeutic Touch has a broad reach. Stress, which responds remarkably well to Therapeutic Touch, underlies psychosomatic illnesses of pandemic proportions. The far-flung symptoms of stress significantly shift many basic physiological systems, altering neurophysiological activity, endocrine and immune system balance, the blood supply and blood pressure, respiratory rate and pattern, and digestion. Studies by Dora Kunz have shown that high stress results in a significantly depressed prana intake and a consequent increase in fatigue. Increases in stress over time open us to changes in the physiological systems, noted above. It may also have decidedly psychological effects, and it is not unusual to see a build-up of unreleased tensions, with a consequent sense of entrapment and ennui. If prolonged, this state of irresolution can rapidly lead to confusion, anxiety, and, in the extreme, to depression.

Therapeutic Touch Skills for Chronic Fatigue Syndrome

The stress scenario is similar to the symptomatic profile of chronic fatigue syndrome (CFS), a current disorder that has grown to epidemic proportions. Chronic fatigue syndrome has a strange history that links it to the Epstein-Barr virus prevalent during the 1970s and '80s, and also to infectious mononucleosis, whose public recognition stretches back to the 1950s at least. The symptoms of both illnesses make those of chronic fatigue syndrome sound like "déjà-vu, all over again." The symptoms of CFS are insidious and do not seem to be of much significance in themselves. Frequently, there are several little things that are hardly noticed in the early stages: headache, upper respiratory infections, recurring sore throat, sleep disturbances, daytime low-grade fever, and generalized muscle and joint pain. In the background is a growing sense of increasing fatigue that seems to provoke bouts of irritability and mood swings. The mounting sense of fatigue is a constant companion and an incessant source of high-grade stress. Intestinal problems come to the forefront of attention, and lymph-node swellings may be noticed—the discoveries driving up the level of anxiety. There may be temporary memory loss and depression. To the person ill with chronic fatigue syndrome, it seems as though it will never go away, as though it is you, yourself, your self-image. The ruminations of the utterly fatigued are familiar: "Who am I? I am sick and tired. Always sick and tired. That is my past history, and my future. I am sick and tired of being sick and tired. But that is me; it is who I am."

How would we begin to help? The most honest answer would be: slowly and thoughtfully. As the symptoms of chronic fatigue syndrome are reviewed, we are impressed that, although they appear commonplace, they indicate that major body systems have become increasingly destabilized, reserve energies have been drained, and recuperative abilities appear overwhelmed. Moreover, there is neither a "bug" to blame nor a "magic-bullet" treatment to prescribe. A cause for caution is that persistent fatigue can be a significant symptom in a host of disorders: anemia, thyroid disorders, autoimmune disorders, neurological dysfunctions, chronic infection, depressive states, and malignancies. In addition, several trigger factors have been cited—magnesium deficiency, hypoglycemia, food intolerance, and yeast infections (Lewis, 1996). This is where the "hard work" of Therapeutic Touch gets personally defined for the Therapeutic Touch therapist, and the inner work of Therapeutic Touch is acknowledged as a priceless ally.

To begin to analyze this problem, there are at least two things I firmly would not do. Chronic Fatigue Syndrome is admittedly a complicated and multifaceted problem, and so I would not presume to "hack it" alone. Even a brief review will indicate that we are seeing in the spread of symptoms a disarray that touches every observable aspect of the healee. Primary physical symptoms are indicated by the persistent headache, muscle and joint pains, and digestive disturbances. Emotional problems are indicated by sleep disturbances, increasing irritability that can progress to anxiety states and depression. Confusion in the use of intellectual faculties is indicated by an inability to concentrate, the ever-present state of weariness, where he or she is "too tired to think" and easily slips into a restive sense of ennui. In addition, there is a lessening access to spiritual unfoldment as a loss of self-confidence deepens and is coupled to a concomitant sense of loss of meaning in life; all too frequently, stark indications come to light of an increasing loss of ability to intimately relate to others and a growing sense of encroaching isolation.

Through referral or in consultation, I would bring in competent persons from other healing modalities. I would emphasize that our goals for the healee must converge, and ask them to work with me as a team to meet the healee's needs. At the least, I would include: persons who do acupuncture and massage; those who could teach the healee how to do meditation and proper ventilatory exercises, such as pranayamas; and either a naturopathic or a homeopathic physician. I would suggest the best practitioners available because, as should be obvious, there is very little room for mediocrity in healing. I would advise a preliminary period of three weeks of treatment, to be followed by a consensual evaluation on the effects of the program, the healee being the major participant in the evaluation. If warranted, I would then propose a second three-week period of treatment, at the end of which we would reevaluate the program and consider long-term goals.

Secondly, I would not do the suggestions of Therapeutic Touch skills, listed in table 3, all at the same time. I would begin by doing them lightly and for short periods of time over the first three sessions. This would give me ample time to get an in-depth understanding of the healee's individual vital-energy field dynamics and its reactions to Therapeutic Touch. Then, continuing to see the healee as much as three times a week, I would go into depth in progressive stages. I would suggest that the healee keep a journal during this period, which I would review with the her or him for the first five or ten minutes of each session. My experience has been that these few minutes give me precious opportunities for insight into the healee as an individual, and I can then custom-tailor the Therapeutic Touch session to meet spoken or implied needs. I would draw up a flow sheet for these first sessions to help keep me on track. The schedule would include the appropriate Therapeutic Touch (TT) skills, as noted in table 3.

It has to be kept in mind that the information in table 3, below, is not a prescription; at best it is an indication of several major aspects of the problem that have to be considered during the Therapeutic Touch sessions. The ultimate determiner of what should go into the rebalancing phase is the individualized assessment of each healee's vital-energy field. Also, the mating of selected Therapeutic Touch skills to selected symptoms when they are separated from a considered opinion about other intervening factors is simply not the way to go. Above all else, it is imperative to keep in mind that we are trying to treat "the whole person." To do this, of course, we must first have some concept of what that term means.

Toward Understanding the "Whole Person"

From personal experience, I would suggest that you practice centering your consciousness and gaining an objective view of the Therapeutic Touch interaction as it unfolds by using, for example, the "Deep Dee" form to keep track of subtle events. This approach best gives you the confidence that a glimpse of the healee as a "whole person" will be perceived clearly, with his or her unique mix of abilities, disabilities, and potential for therapeutic change. Of course, that glimpse stands ready to be rectified or enlarged; much depends on the reach of individual insight as the interaction proceeds, and the Therapeutic Touch therapist's inner work clarifies his or her understanding of the healee.

Acknowledging the Inner Self

A maintained state of centered consciousness is the focal point around which the practice of Therapeutic Touch revolves, and the source from which it gains its power. Therefore, what you as therapist are trying to do is reach beyond the usual perspective of things-as-they-are, and attempt to align with the perspective of your personal inner self. In this outreach to actualize personal potentials for insightful and creative healing in the service of those in need, you perceive for yourself the power for change, as that change is reflected

TABLE 3

List of Therapeutic Touch Skills Appropriate for Initial Sessions re: Chronic Fatigue Syndrome Symptoms

TT Skills	Symptoms	Primary Site:
Directing vital energies	Depleted prana	solar plexus chakra (over adrenal sites)
	Recurring sore throat	lymphatic chains
	Depressed immune system	thymus gland
	Toxicity	spleen-liver shunt
	Irritability, anxiety, and depression	heart chakra and solar plexus chakra
Modulating vital energies	Fatigue	*Golden Yellow to: spleen and solar plexus chakras and interface massage at neck muscles
	Recurring sore throat	lymphatic chains and thymus gland
	Need for psychological support	*Rose to:heart chakra
	Lymph-node swelling	*Blue to: major lymph nodes
	Intestinal problems	solar plexus chakra
	Muscle and joint pain	involved sites
	Headache	internal carotids, neck muscles, and solar plexus chakra
	Sleep disturbances	throat and heart chakras
	Toxicity	*Green to: spleen and liver
	Temporary memory loss	*Violet to: heart chakra
	Spiritual detachment	all upper chakras
Unruffling vital energies	Low-grade fever	total body, plus blue modulation
	Muscle and joint pain	at sites involved, and then moving toward extremities
	Emotional problems	heart and solar plexus chakras
	Lymph-node swelling	from lymphatic site toward the extremity

in your own life events and in the quality of your Therapeutic Touch interactions.

The point intended is twofold. Since the evidence of a subtle reflection of your inner life becomes clarified through a committed, centered state of consciousness, and such proposition is supported by events occurring in the everyday happenings of your life, I urge that such occurrence should be acknowledged to yourself, at the least. Secondly, you are then encouraged to go one step further: Recognize that the healee also has an inner self, and act as though that is a reality. In other words, the suggestion is that during the Therapeutic Touch interaction, as you feel yourself deeply centered and in touch with your inner self, you should bring the forces of your intentionality into play and align them with an attempt to communicate mind-to-mind with the inner self of the healee.

Using Intentionality to Access the Inner Self

How you do this is difficult to describe, but the basic steps involve at least two factors. You need a reliable sense of that inner connection as the experience plays through your consciousness and, secondly, and most necessary, you need the ability to translate that comprehension into a clear communication, mind-to-mind, with what you conceive to be a similar state of consciousness in the healee.

The operative words in this instruction are "a clear communication." The actual process is much like what occurs during mental telepathy. However, the motivating force that carries the message is of the greatest importance, for a fleeting sense of the quality of the experience may be all that the healee's conscious mind is able to pick up, and to become aware of the other's base emotions in regard to one's personal well-being can be disconcerting.

The inner work that you are doing in this mind-to-mind communication is a message to the inner self of the healee, perhaps preceded by a simple, silent, mind-to-mind greeting or acknowledgement of presence. Assistance in the healing engagement is then asked of that aspect of the healee. There may be no way of knowing what the healee's private agenda about his or her illness is; however, properly done, there is nothing about the attempt that will do harm and, therefore, it is worth a try. In those instances where conjoint and cooperative efforts work on behalf of the needs of the healee, the healing can be effective and surprisingly rapid. This effect is not magical; rather, it reinforces the notion that all healing is dependent on self-healing.

Supporting Self-Healing

During the Therapeutic Touch interaction, it is when the rebalancing phase is reached that the skills noted in table 3 are brought into play. At first glance, the symptomatic picture presented by chronic fatigue syndrome appears intimidating. However, if you look at the various suggested Therapeutic Touch skills, and then pay particular attention to the groups of symptoms listed under each skill, you will note that from the point of view of Therapeutic Touch—which is concerned only with the human energies involved in our functions and behaviors, not with medical diagnoses—the symptoms in each group display an intrinsic similarity when they are thought of as functional results of the way the human energy, prana, is moving through the individual. For instance, under the heading, "Directing vital energies," all of the symptoms indicate a need to replenish, stimulate, or detoxify depleted pranic systems and to assure that they remain in a balanced state. This begins to give you a hint about what is systemically awry in the pranic flows, and will also suggest how these aberrations can be rebalanced in a holistic fashion in which the healee plays the leading self-healing role.

To assure that process, the convention has been developed over time of allowing the healee—who usually has been affected by the rapid and profound relaxation response during the Therapeutic Touch session—to lie down or to sit quietly for ten or fifteen minutes at the end of the session. It is not unusual for the person to fall asleep. You can encourage and facilitate this by covering the healee with a light blanket, for, of all the natural functions of the body, the greatest amount of regeneration and self-healing occurs during sleep.

The epitome of the Therapeutic Touch process can be seen to be at work in the microcosm of this example: You strive to fulfill a compassionate concern for the needs of the healee and, therefore, stretch and exercise your inner faculties in the quest of a conscious understanding and engagement in the healing interaction. The healee, secure in the human support system provided by you, opens him- or herself to the healing process by relaxing, perhaps sleeping, and thereby giving opportunity for the depths of the unconscious to join forces with the resources of the inner self on behalf of his or her wellbeing. For the healee, it marks a period of appreciation of the capacity for self-healing, and an opportunity for the acceptance of the therapeutic changes the healing will offer. In addition, and importantly for you as Therapeutic Touch therapist, it is an opportunity for the realization of your inner potentials in the cause of helping others; for cognizance of the self-growth that occurs in the process; for a grasp of the inner work that makes the experience meaningful; and for a not-to-be-forgotten chance for personal insight in grappling with the question, *"Why do I want to be healer?"*

THE NATURAL
THERAPEUTIC TOUCH
CONNECTION

Some people can be quite specific about the chakras they use under particular circumstances. When I was a child, trees were my first friends. As I got older, I felt I could have meaningful exchanges of thought with them using what I then considered to be different parts of my body, such as my throat. It wasn't until I became deeply involved in the intentional use of chakras in healing, however, that I began to appreciate the specificity of consciousness of the different chakras, and to realize that there is a direct relationship between the species of tree I communicated with and the chakra that was used.

I thought that this was a personal, fanciful notion. However, a few years ago I had the distinct joy and privilege of spending some time with one of the most powerful and well-known witch doctors in Africa, Credo Vusa' Mazulu Mutwa. He is also well known for the quality of his artistic and literary abilities (Mutwa, 1969). He had eight of his students demonstrate for me what they had learned from him and answer my questions. Later, as our discussion deepened, Credo and I found that we had several experiences in common in reference to healing and to the teaching of healing. We discussed the development of sensitivities to all life forms by persons studying healing, and the correlation between the chakra one uses in communication with specific tree species. One of my students taped the conversation, which took place in Soweto, a village outside of Johannesburg, and the following is a section of the transcription. We had been speaking about the effect human emotions have on plants.

D: What I would very much like to ask, sir, is: Do you, yourself, communicate with plants and trees? Do you find that you are able to communicate with various plants and trees by using different parts of your body? For instance, I found with the trees I lived with in the woodlands of Northeastern United States, where most of the trees are hardwood, that when I communicated with them, I did so with this part of me, just beyond or outside the throat.

C: AH-HA! Yes, professor.

D: I am very anxious to speak to you of this, sir. In the far Western part of my country, we have several very large trees, that are many, many years old, the sequoias.

C: Yes, the sequoias; I've been there.

D: Yes, in the Muir Woods in the Bay area, for instance. To my surprise, when I am there and I sit and meditate and try to get in touch with the sequoias, then I find that I communicate from up here, from the top of my head, from what in Sanskrit is called the *sahasrara*, or crown, chakra.

C: (Laughter).

D: And when I am in the desert and I try to get in touch with the tall cactus . . . then, again to my surprise, I find that I communicate through here, through the solar plexus chakra, and obviously from the look on your face, you do too. (Laughter). This is what I would like to share with you.

C: You see, professor, let us say, now I am talking with one of those trees which grow near here. I find there is a slight cold in my feet, around about here in my legs (pointing to certain secondary chakras in the legs). The more deeply we communicate, the more the slight cold rises. The same, exactly the same as you feel. This tree is not indigenous to Africa. We use this (other) tree for the treatment of rheumatism. Now, when I try to talk to that one, its spirit comes not to me through the body, but through the top of the head. Now, I thought I was the only one who felt this, but I see others do too.

As a result of that meeting, Credo had a necklace made which he blessed and gave to me, and he also gave me a name. In Zulu, it is Uyezwa, which I was told translates to "She Who Understands." I look upon this name as a kind of credentializing. It stirs within me the realization that these experiences are real and have a validity to which others can attest.

The "Deep Dee"

How do we do more than catch a fleeting glimpse of these personal knowledges? How do we really, really know that these inner experiences are, indeed, real? Recognizing that reality is relative to values and perspectives, it is possible nevertheless to conjure up a sounding board of reality that will appease even the rage for stark pragmatism that structures reality for our time. Such a reference is the "Deep Dee" forms.

The "Deep Dee" forms were developed primarily as a hedge against the major enemies of Therapeutic Touch, the four bad dragons: impulse, fantasy, exaggeration, and wishful thinking. These destructive dragons need to be under constant vigilance, because they can be inserted too easily and thoughtlessly into the healing act by those who are casual about their responsibilities to the healee and to society. They can make a mindless farce out of a sensitive interaction that initially intends only to be helpful—and these dragons can be decidedly harmful. The antidote is to provide a means for recording experiences as they happen, in the context, idiom, and nuance of the moment, and that is where the "Deep Dee" is helpful.

The name "Deep Dee" was coined by a friend, Jeanne, who had been a feisty journalist before being diagnosed with multiple sclerosis. One day, in describing the in-depth reach of the Therapeutic Touch session we had just completed, she jokingly dubbed the experience "the Deep Dee," and the expression stuck. Later, I was challenged to verbalize my inner experiences during the Therapeutic Touch interaction. As a result, the forms, now known as the "Deep Dee," were developed in an attempt to objectify my own experience and to provide students with a simple guide, designed to help them recollect their own inner experiences with the Therapeutic Touch process.

The "Deep Dee" form seeks to elicit several aspects of the inner work performed by the therapist during the Therapeutic Touch interaction with the healee. "The 'Deep Dee' Form, Part I" (see chapter 3, p. 18) is concerned with how we perceive the process of Therapeutic Touch during the Therapeutic Touch interaction. "The 'Deep Dee', Part II" is reproduced below. It is an extension of Part I and seeks to capture how we use our inner sensitivities to relate to barely perceptible vital-energy functionings. The purpose of the "Deep Dee" form is to provide a simple method for recording experiences that well up from deep within the Therapeutic Touch therapist, so that they can be analyzed at a later time, and personal strategies can be fine-tuned to trace these experiences to their source. When this conscious contact with the source of your human energies is realized, you begin to understand with greater surety how to use them expertly in augmenting the healing process. The major contribution the "Deep Dee" makes is that it helps you separate out the conscious, objective experiences that can be articulated with some ease, from the interior, subjective "listening" experienced when you attend to the dynamic expressions of the vital-energy systems. These latter considerably challenge your ability to describe them. They are most often recollected in metaphoric expressions, if you are able to translate that subtle experience into words at all, and usually they remain as an impression, rather than as a true knowing. The worth of the exercise is that it captures for you the far-flung congeries of your personal knowledge as they arise spontaneously during the Therapeutic Touch session, and sequesters them for later analysis and clarification.

The Intentional Use of the Chakras

Chakras can be thought of as nonphysical, two-way converter stations, where psychic forces and physical functions merge into, and penetrate, each other. For example, they act as focal points within which forces of the localized universal psychodynamic field are tempered and gel into form as characteristic psychological expressions of the individual's physical being.

How can we best get in touch with these points of entry that are so necessary to our human functioning? These forces directly account for the vital characteristics that distinguish us as human beings—the spectrum of the feeling-thinking continuum we call emotions. There are, of course, the outward expressions of these emotions; however, once expressed they fade rapidly from memory, and not many in the Western cultures are given to self-analysis of sufficient depth to trace back these emotions to their source in the psyche.

However, the autonomic nervous system (ANS), which is sensitive to the feeling-thinking moment, does leave its physiological imprint long enough to make a conscious impression. As a classic example, we know when we are frightened because our hands are sweaty, our heart rate is unusually rapid, and our guts are heaving. It is the memory of such instantaneous, but nevertheless second-hand, effects that provides us with a link to the recognition, if not understanding, of these dynamic sources of our humanness—the chakras. We find that if we trace back these ANS signals, we get a good idea of the fullness of the emotion, some understanding of how the related chakras function, and an inkling of how they can be tapped.

In healing, meaning comes through the process of the healing itself, the experiential knowledge providing both context and depth to the understanding. As noted, these clues are frequently expressed to the consciousness through specific physiological changes and deep-gut feelings. Awareness also arises from ill-defined and emotionally laden impressions that well up from the unconscious and from little understood deep-brain structures. Often they are encrypted in metaphor and symbol, occasionally to be enlightened by dream or hunch, true insight or intuition. These functions can be called upon in our quest to understand the nature of our own chakras, and Part 2 of the "Deep Dee," below, is designed to help in this inquiry.

EXPLORATIONS OF THE SELF 14

"Listening" to the "Deep Dee," Part 2

Expression of the Chakra:	How I Am Accessing the Chakra:
	Prompting: Interpretation:

A. Love (heart chakra):

B. Peace (throat chakra):

C. Compassion (integration
   of heart and throat chakras):

   Associated Ideas:

   Self-evaluation:

Suggestions for Using the "Deep Dee," Part 2

Self-Exploration of the Heart Chakra

Begin by centering quietly for a minute or two, and then think of someone you truly love. As you send love to that person, be aware of what is happening to you, both physically and nonphysically. What love itself feels like was explored in the "Deep Dee," Part I (see chapter 3, p. 18). In this exercise, you are trying to get beyond that initial perception and, using the feeling of love as it flows through you as a basis for your identification of an expression of the heart chakra, trying to trace those particular vibes back to their source at the heart chakra itself. Ask yourself: Where is that particular feeling tone coming from? How are its forces working through me? What vital-energy clues are being offered about the essential nature of this loveflow as I follow it to its source? Maintain your sense of that loveflow and explore more deeply this state of consciousness. Do not structure the experience with your own expectations; use your consciousness as a sensitive probe and allow it to tell you its own story. Keep pen and paper nearby and jot down a note or two about what is occurring. Try to quietly maintain your state of centered consciousness, but do not exert effort; go with the loveflow, and attentively "listen."

I start by centering my consciousness. As I close my eyes to more clearly access the feeling of love, I am aware of a strong, uplifting, outward flow. Caught up in this powerful outpouring of feeling, it is not difficult to construct a thoughtform of my beloved in my mindspace, and it happens very quickly: Suddenly, there is this light, beautiful sense of presence. I feel a sweet at-oneness with him, and his presence gives me pleasure. Soft and tender feelings of affection for him arise within me. I notice that this gentle mood is generalized, and it is easy to send thoughts of tenderness to others as well. Love seems to have no bounds as it wells up within me. It percolates effortlessly through me, and I learn to modulate the ceaseless loveflow so that its intensity does not overwhelm me.

It is only after a while that I realize that the crown chakra seems to be involved also. My supposition is that the crown chakra is involved in the experience because of the conscious construction of the thoughtform. A momentary break in concentration entices me to play with the thoughtform. I realize that it is an imagery, rather than a true visualization, for I can make the thoughtform shift at will in whatever way I wish. In that moment I am also aware that I have lost my conscious connection to the heart chakra, and have to start from the beginning again. But the second time around it is easier to recapture the experience of the loveflow, and with renewed perseverance I trace it back to its source as a major function of the heart chakra. I can maintain that identity in full consciousness for only a little while, but memory helps me recapture the sense of it.

Self-Exploration of the Throat Chakra

I will now elicit the functions of the throat chakra by using the concept of peace. I begin, as always, by centering. As the idea of peace courses through me, I note that its outward-seeking flow is decidedly goal-oriented. This swelling, but nonetheless tranquil, tide is suffused with a surge of altruism, a will to the good, and a feeling of serenity and quietude. The atmosphere it creates is permissive and protective, and a sense of freedom from fear and anxiety pervades. Within its refuge, a privileged opportunity for unrestricted, spontaneous feelings and creative thought seems at hand. This coherent, vital flow representative of the essence of peace is consistent with my most satisfying self-imaging of it. I feel in balance, serene, and, in my mind's eye, as I step gently upon Earth again, I walk in beauty.

Thus grounded, I realize that my throat muscles are relaxed, even the little muscles around my eyes and my ears are relaxed. The nature of the moment itself is stress-free, the vibratory level of its rhythm is softly modulated and reflects a sense of unperturbed calmness that permeates my entire being. It is as though a resonant note had been gently sounded, and its faint, melodious resounding continues to echo in the background of my consciousness. It finally carries its vibratory experience effortlessly beyond my ability to be aware, but leaves me with a lingering sense of its harmonic presence. My most vivid impression is that the throat chakra's major capability is the expert integration of several aspects of deeply felt emotions, lending them coherence and giving them living expression.

Integrating the Chakras: A Self-Exploration of Compassion

I now go on to explore within myself the concept of compassion. I begin by consciously aligning myself with my clearest sense of inner self, and simultaneously observing closely what seems to be happening within my vital-energy field as I think about compassion.

It is easiest to report on the physiological correlates, those physical effects that occur at the same time as I focus on compassion and that may have a direct relation to its process. First noticed are my respirations, which become deeper and fuller. My muscles are relaxed, I feel calm and comfortable, and I have a sense of well-being.

Emotion wells up in my throat, which feels full for a moment. Simultaneously, my heart energies "go out" to the individual or people for whom I have this concern. In particular, my upper chakras feel coordinated or in dynamic alignment; the flow of vital energies is steady, strong, and outgoing, emerging from both my heart and my throat chakras, the two in faultless synchrony.

As I focus on the object of my compassion, a felt shift in consciousness occurs, and I visualize with some clarity a figure or a symbol. As this occurs, the visualization seems to coalesce and form just beyond my face, at about the level of my lower forehead, while my eyes themselves are either open or closed. That is, the eyes themselves seem to have little to do with these mind pictures.

My sense of it is that I have some help at this time—probably my emotions more clearly configurate—but it is only an impression, which I cannot articulate fully or well. I also have the impression that my crown chakra is engaged in this event—not as an upsurge of energy, but rather as a distinct presence that is both within and beyond me at the same time. I am not aware of time passing, but I do know when I am no longer working with the energies of compassion. At that time, however, I have a good idea of how, or if, I can be of help, and I find that appropriate creative strategies of Therapeutic Touch easily come to mind.

I am left with the impression, which has become clearer over time, that the act of attempting (struggling!) to work consciously with more than one chakra at a time and trying to understand the vital-energetic relationships between them, seems to have had a synergistic effect on the reliability of several subtle functions, such as intuition and mind-to-mind communication. I see some evidence of this effect in my Therapeutic Touch practices today and in my daily social relationships. For instance, increasingly there is immediate cognizance of the implications of my assessment of the healee's vital-energy field during the Therapeutic Touch interaction, and this insight proves to be correct at a later date.

In conjunction with doing the "Deep Dee" analyses, I also recommend keeping a journal of how these analyses affect the inner work of your own Therapeutic Touch practices. Report on feelings and thoughts, but also keep a record of impressions and images that pop into your mind, moods and inner promptings that drive you, and dreams, particularly if they are repetitive or lucid, and especially if they are recalled during the day. Be also aware of metaphors you use and note coincidences that occur. I push my intuition by following its insight every time I hear its quiet voice. By following up on how the incident finally turned out, I learn how to be more discriminative in judgment, and I begin to recognize the distinctive signatures that mark true intuition and distinguish it from mere hunch.

I recommend that you read your current journal in one sitting about every six weeks and, as objectively as you can, evaluate your experiences. Encourage a healthy sensitivity to your own path by noting inner changes that are occurring in your daily routine, in your life circumstances, and in your insights about yourself and others. Then ask yourself some direct questions: What are these changes telling me? How has my self-concept changed, and is it warranted? What have I learned about my inner work that will help me in my healing work?

Consciousness-Raising in the Service of Healing

Healing is not just about fixing the "owie." It is about stabilizing the panic-stricken, reaching through heavy veils of loneliness, providing sanctuary for those who are frightened, and sharing a healing moment with those moving through final transition. The beauty of knowing how to access deeply your own chakras on command is the ability to respond with confidence to the needs of such people even when nothing else seems to help; to know how to intelligently and compassionately use your vital-energy field as a human support system for those in need; and to touch them in a manner few have been touched before.

For you as Therapeutic Touch therapist, this active inner search to seek out the essential being of your own chakras is an intentional act of consciousness-raising. To embark on this search out of compassion for others makes a powerful ally of this exploration of the deep self. It is important to keep in mind that in attempting to experientially understand your own chakras, you are searching for a point of entry into a little-known domain of which we have become cognizant only recently. We are not only trying to become more fully self-aware, which is a basic distinguishing feature of our human nature, but we are also trying to plumb to the core the many aspects of consciousness of which we are heir.

Experience will convince you that even turning your attention in this direction acts to stir your mind-set and significantly rouse your consciousness from the usual soporific state where many of us indolently dwell. However, it is when you resolutely seek out your own roots in the inner recesses of your mind so that you can better help others that there occurs a vibrant coupling of irresistible forces: a thirsting quest for your own unique grasp of wisdom joined with a passion for relieving the suffering of others. This purposeful bonding accelerates and refines the process marvelously, for in this consciousness-raising in the service of helping or healing others, the inner work of the chakra complex acts synergistically on the many aspects of the individual's consciousness and achieves significantly more for both the Therapeutic Touch therapist and the healee than either act could accomplish alone.

Thus, for several reasons, the "Deep Dee" analysis can become a useful and important exercise in the mature practice of Therapeutic Touch. The power of healing rests at least as much upon what you, yourself, are as a dynamic being as on what you do, for the subtle structure of your own vital-energy field is the medium for your healing message. Therefore, do not let the opportunity pass by to engage your most human capabilities in a most humane way. Be adamant in your quest and be open to creative implementation in how you go about it. If, in your attempt to learn about the heart chakra, you have no one from whom to experience love, adopt an animal—perhaps two to keep each other company—and open yourself to their very natural, powerful expressions of love. These furry and feathered "other nations" (Beston, 1928) are excellent teachers. If you need help learning about your throat chakra, join a choral group that has a very good musical director. The many members of the choral group will cover for you if you don't sing well, and in the meantime you have an opportunity to objectively regard your throat chakra at work. As previously noted, there is a strong analogy between modulating your voice and modulating the vital-energy field during the Therapeutic Touch rebalancing. Here are some final suggestions for your consideration: If you are trying to learn to communicate mind-to-mind, seek out a place in nature where wild animals and birds pass by (a few squirrels or sparrows in a park work fine). Center yourself and, even if there seems to be no one about at the time, within your mind, put out a call to the two-leggeds and the four-leggeds. If you are successful, the response will be unforgettable. As you gain some proficiency, try this with the fluid energies of moving, living waters, and the telluric energies of the "Rainbow Serpent" sleeping in large rock forms, and the very different, explicit intelligence of ancient trees. Don't be content to talk with them; exchange ideas and record your impressions. Of course, in certain circles this may make you indubitably certifiable, but it's so much fun!

For other "out-of-this-world" experiences, try Explorations of the Self 15, "Doin' My ET-TT: The Venusian Encounter," below. Before doing so, you may want to review Explorations of the Self 3. "On Being Present: An Exercise in Intentionality" (see chapter 1, p. 13).

EXPLORATIONS OF THE SELF 15

Doin' My ET-TT: The Venusian Encounter

Note: In the Therapeutic Touch assessment, we could say that we are laying a base for a new kind of social communication, for, with only the use of hand and other chakras, we obtain information from the healee's vital-energy field. Exploration of the Self 15 is an exercise in using your chakras to communicate with another person, one who happens to be an ET (extraterrestial being) from the planet Venus.

"Doin' My ET-TT: A Venusian Encounter" requires pairs of people working together. One of each pair will play the role of an Earthling named Harry the Humble Healer, and the other person will play the role of Re-La-Eh (strong accent on the last syllable). Re-La-Eh is the word "healer" spelled backward, and she/he is a Venusian.

Ideally, groups of four people will do this exploration at the same time. In that case, each group will break up into two pairs, so that A will work with B, and C will work with D. In each pair, one will be Harry the Humble Healer, and the other person will be Re-La-Eh. After the exploration is completed and all have had an opportunity to record the experience in their notes, they change roles, without sharing their experiences, and repeat the exploration. At the end of this exploration, and after all notes have been recorded but not yet shared, both pairs change partners so that A is now with C, and B with D, and they repeat the exploration.

To make full use of the time, there can be a further exchange of partners so that A pairs up with D, and B pairs with C, and the exploration can be repeated one more time.

Materials

Paper and pen.

Procedure

1. To begin, each pair will decide who will be Harry the Humble

Healer and who will be Re-La-Eh, the Venusian. When this has been decided, both center for a few moments.

2. Directions for Harry:

Imagine that you have always wanted to have an out-of-body experience. Tonight your wish has been granted, and you succeed in going to the planet Venus. You navigate the vaporous atmospheres easily and acclimate instantly. You land and wander around, taking in the sights. As you turn a corner, you come face-to-face with a Venusian, Re-La-Eh.

You are not intimidated by the Venusian, but you find that you don't understand the Venusian language, nor does Re-La-Eh understand what you are saying.

Working on the assumption that Venusians have chakras, you use your chakras to convey a message to Re-La-Eh. Nod to Re-La-Eh when you are ready to send the message. Send the message on your exhalations, directing your breath to your appropriate chakra at the same time.

3. Directions for Re-La-Eh:

When you see Harry nod, do a Therapeutic Touch assessment on Harry. Go through Harry's entire vital-energy field at a moderate pace, without stopping. Then reassess any region of the field you want to check. Write down your impressions of the message Harry was trying to convey. Don't exchange information at this time.

4. Harry will also write down the message he or she was trying to communicate, and any impressions of the experience.

5. When this exploration has been completed, change partners according to the schedule as outlined above. This will give each member of the group three opportunities to give and receive messages.

6. After the last exploration has been completed, all four meet as a group and discuss all of the experiences. Picking up the exact words of Harry's message will be unusual, but that is secondary.

Of prime importance will be Re-La-Eh's account of her/his inner work in trying to pick up Harry's communication. As you discuss your experiences, in particular note similarities and differences in your experiences, and novel or unexpected approaches to the problems of extraterrestrial communications.

The Empowerment of Compassion

I frequently have wondered at the power of compassion. It is by no means a survival skill, and I am in awe that it has continued to surge in the hearts of humankind over the millennia. Why? One answer might be that that is how we are supposed to relate to one another—perhaps it is in Nature's best interests that we exercise this most humane of all human traits toward other beings. Perhaps the success of evolution is not so much a matter *that* we survive, as *how* we survive.

The point has been made in earlier chapters that compassion is a necessary background for the therapist's use of Therapeutic Touch practices. It is not merely that without compassion as the motivating factor, the practice of Therapeutic Touch is in jeopardy of being nothing but a power play. It is also a subjectively testable fact that it is the dynamic nature of compassion that provides the opportunity to plunge into the farther reaches of our own consciousness, access our finest capabilities, and thus bring the wonder of the healing act into being for someone in need. It is, indeed, this irrepressible passion to help others that supplies the remarkable energetic thrust necessary for the decisive quantum leap that distinguishes the vitalizing state of healing from the debilitating state of illness. The integrative force we know as compassion shapes a path for universal healing energies to flow through our being, and it is through the experiential knowledge that attends that outpouring that we get an opportunity, in the healing moment, to acknowledge the reality of our inner self.

During the Therapeutic Touch engagement, this acknowledgment follows directly from the assessment phase, which is itself empowered by the state of centered consciousness maintained throughout the Therapeutic Touch interaction. It is during the assessment that we perceive information directly from the healee's vital-energy field, and these bits of information then provide us with a structural framework or perspective of personal knowledge as the Therapeutic Touch process flows through us. As this healing enactment continues, the process deeply engages us and—for a moment and if we are duly aware—we have a fleeting recognition of having been touched by a complex of universal healing energies in which both healer and healee hold common ground. It is then that we intuit that it is not only healer and healee who are engaged in the healing act, but also some "X" factor has resounded through the healing moment in a manner that is transpersonal and, frequently, transverbal.

We may also perceive at that time that Therapeutic Touch is in fact a discipline—in the sense of it being a self-disciplined search to learn the inner work that evokes the depths of the Therapeutic Touch practice and makes of it a lifestyle. It is also a discipline in the sense that Therapeutic Touch is a distinctive branch of healer education as a contemporary interpretation of several ancient healing practices, practices that are structured under a primary assumption that healing itself is a natural potential.

Therapeutic Touch as a Transpersonal Act

You can now clearly see that the act of centering that empowers Therapeutic Touch is not a passive act, but is an active exploration of the inner self and a knowledgeable use of its facets in the inner work of Therapeutic Touch. In the process, Therapeutic Touch emerges as a transpersonal act as you, under the persistent urges of compassionate concern, gain confidence—permitting the higher orders of self to lead the way—and see the gratifying response to such trust. It is here that you as Therapeutic Touch therapist fully "come out of the closet," transcend cultural biases, and allow the convictions of your inner life to interact with the outer, more socialized, ego-centered self, the persona, and to permeate its daily activities.

In the throes of this translation of conviction into deed, there is a dawning awareness of the unitary nature of that inner self, as the experiential knowledge garnered during the healing act clarifies the recognition of potential common bonds of consciousness between all living beings. Our strivings in making Therapeutic Touch a conscious act quicken our own potential for intuition and insight. Appreciating the uncommonly fine edge these qualities lend to the healing skills, we voluntarily self-control the stability of our psychic forces and transmute unbridled impulse into considered action in the interest of meeting the needs of the healee. Aided by this potent shift in perception, there follows a compelling change in worldview and a subsequent decided reshaping of lifestyle.

Thus, we see that healing, processed through unobstructed acts of compassion, brings into your life a unique energetic, the finer energies of the higher orders of the self. These harbingers of the inner self have been accessed through the conscious exercise of the upper chakras during the healing act itself. It is as these personal knowledges are acquired by the Therapeutic Touch therapist, and are actively engaged in the practice of Therapeutic Touch, that this compassion-born interaction, itself, provides the opportunity of accessing the transpersonal. In this way you gain entry to inner, subjective sources of guidance and inspiration, and your personality acquires the stability to subject these insights to tests verified by the inner work. In the final analysis, it is these tests provided by your inner work that answer the persistent query: *"Why do I want to be healer?"*

9

THERAPEUTIC TOUCH AS A SOCIAL FORCE

Therapeutic Touch in the Wider Community

Deplaning in Edmonton, Canada, to present a paper at an international conference, I quickly sought the distinctive banner of the conference's hospitality table where I was to meet the person designated to drive me to the hotel. Following directions, I approached the ramp leading to the baggage claim area and noticed a woman descending several feet ahead of me. At the base of the ramp I could see the hospitality table, behind which sat two women. I shifted my briefcase and carry-on bag to descend the ramp.

I hadn't taken more than a half-dozen steps when I saw the woman ahead of me trip and suddenly lunge forward into a full-body fall. I ran to help her, noting at the same time that the two women at the hospitality desk rapidly rose to go to her aid. They reached the fallen woman before I did, and as I approached I heard one say to the other, "She's hurt! Do Therapeutic Touch, quickly!" Realizing she was right, I obediently put down my briefcase and bag, slid out of my raincoat, and turned to do Therapeutic Touch to the injured woman—to find that the two hospitality women were already at work on her, exchanging information about their individual assessments and planning their rebalancing strategies.

I stood aside and watched the two women engrossed in their work. It took me a moment or two to realize that not only were they doing very well without me, but they also didn't even recognize me or my relation to the founding of Therapeutic Touch. If I hadn't realized it before, I now clearly understood that Therapeutic Touch had taken on a life of its own and would get along very well with or without me in the coming years.

In the twenty-four years since Dora Kunz and I introduced Therapeutic Touch, it has developed rapidly and has been very helpful as a healing modality. Besides the intensive studies and theory development in which Dora and I have been engaged, at this writing there have been twenty-seven doctoral dissertations on Therapeutic Touch accepted at universities in the United States; eighteen postdoctoral researches on Therapeutic Touch have been reported out; and innumerable clinical studies and master's degree theses have been completed. To date, I have taught Therapeutic Touch to over 43,000 professional persons in the health field in addition to several thousand laypersons, and over the years our students have probably taught again as many in their own private practices.

There have been a large number of magazine articles and several books on Therapeutic Touch, and many commentaries on all the major channels of electronic media in the United States and Canada. Therapeutic Touch has also received considerable attention elsewhere in the world, including very active and continuing dialogues internationally on the Internet by way of "America On-line," "Prodigy," and other on-line services.

As has been called to my attention, Therapeutic Touch has historically been the first healing modality to be an integral part of a fully accredited university curriculum. At present, Therapeutic Touch has been taught at more than one hundred colleges and universities in the United States, and has been taught in seventy-five foreign countries. One of the courses in the United States is a graduate-level seminar for biology majors. The professor tells me that Therapeutic Touch provides the model for inquiry into the nature of biology of the twenty-first century.

Professional literature on Therapeutic Touch has been so extensive that since 1988 it has been consistently cited on Medline, the computerized retrieval system for literature significant to the health professions. Therapeutic Touch has also found its way into the popular literature. For instance, two days ago, Neila, a Therapeutic Touch practitioner sent me copy of Michael Palmer's current bestseller, *Extreme Measures.* On page 100, Palmer is writing about "a crack E.R. nurse," Terri Dillard, and says, ". . . her massage and Therapeutic Touch often had patients diagnosed or actually cured before a physician even entered the room." (My comment: "Michael, Michael; you DREAM....but, it has happened!")

Therapeutic Touch in the Family

In 1985, I completed a report based on funded research on marital relationships. In the protocol, I had taught husbands how to do Therapeutic Touch to their pregnant wives during the third trimester, when the fetuses were six-to-nine months in utero, and the husbands continued the Therapeutic Touch until the birth of the child. The study was successful, with no untoward reactions to the Therapeutic Touch practices.

It was so enjoyable for the couples that several dozen in the experimental group continued doing Therapeutic Touch within the family after the birth of their children. Therapeutic Touch flourished within the family, with family members doing Therapeutic Touch to one another instead of reaching for an aspirin. In several families Therapeutic Touch was incorporated into the family daily life. For instance, when the breadwinner would return from work at the end of the day, as an expression of love and concern, a family member would offer that person Therapeutic Touch for its rapid relaxation response ". . . to help him or her escape the raw jungle mind-set of the competitive business world, so that he or she could become human again," as one parent put it. Very rapidly these intrafamily practices were passed on to relatives and friends, and small groups carried it into the community.

Therapeutic Touch as a Social Force

I, myself, did not fully realize how great the demand was for Therapeutic Touch until 1989 when I received two phone calls within days of one another. They were from different parts of the country, but they were both from hospital administrators and both had the same message. They were calling to tell me that their offices were receiving calls from local citizens who were facing hospitalization. In each case, the callers wanted to be assured that Therapeutic Touch was practiced in that hospital so that they could have Therapeutic Touch sessions following the medical procedures. If this assurance could not be given, the callers said, they would seek out another hospital where Therapeutic Touch could be done. Even the second time I heard it, it took me a moment or two to react intelligently. It was only over time that I realized that, with its emphasis on compassion for those in need, and with the personal challenges its inner work presented to the Therapeutic Touch therapist, Therapeutic Touch had become a strong social force. Simultaneously, the move of Therapeutic Touch into the community attracted the enthusiasm of hospice volunteers and staff members. Within two years Therapeutic Touch was being practiced in hospices in both the United States and Canada, where it continues to help many enter a peaceful final transition.

Therapeutic Touch Abroad

Therapeutic Touch has been practiced in many "hot spots" of the world. A lasting memory from a month-long lecture tour in South Africa is the sight of persons of all skin colors practicing Therapeutic Touch on one another. I was told that before peace was invoked by Muhammad Anwar Sadat's visit to Israel, Therapeutic Touch was practiced by both Israelis and Egyptians in the Gaza Strip. During the early 1980s it was introduced into the refugee camps in Thailand and, later, into Cambodia itself. Some of the refugees would join American hospital volunteers doing Therapeutic Touch because it reminded them of their own folk practices.

Therapeutic Touch also has been taught in Ho Chi Minh City, Vietnam. Carolyn and John are two long-time Therapeutic Touch therapists. In a strange crossover of time, but without intentional design, while Carolyn was teaching Therapeutic Touch in Ho Chi Minh City, John was holding Therapeutic Touch sessions for several veterans of the Vietnam War in the back of a bar and grill in New Jersey. Therapeutic Touch has been taught in several regions of China and, when a tourist was injured, it was practiced at the Great Wall itself.

The Reach of Therapeutic Touch in the Americas

Narrowing our scope to the Americas, Therapeutic Touch has been taught in a wide arc above the Arctic Circle in the trading posts of the Northwest Territories in Canada to the United States Public Health Hospital in Kotzebue, Alaska. It has been practiced in the rain forests of Brazil and the grassy pampas of Argentina, and beyond the continent east to Puerto Rico in the Atlantic, and west to Hawaii and to Guam in the Mariana Islands in the Pacific.

Therapeutic Touch in Emergency Situations

Therapeutic Touch has been practiced in many American communities during natural catastrophes, such as among the sandbag crews during the Mississippi floods of 1993; in both the California earthquake and the Montana forest fires the next year; and in the streets following the terrorist bombing in Oklahoma City in 1995. It is being used on exhausted and overexposed persons caught in the floods in Oregon as I write this.

Therapeutic Touch as been used in everyday emergencies by emergency medical technicians who ride the ambulances and the air rescue heliocopters; firefighters; trauma personnel at the scene of automobile and other accidents; emergency-room staffs; lifeguards at beaches; and ski patrols. The patrols use it on the ski slopes particularly for fractures, because its reliable and rapid relaxation response gives them the opportunity to set the bone and immobilize it before transporting the injured person down the mountain.

Under much less organized conditions, Marsha and Gretchen, two graduate students learning about Therapeutic Touch, were hiking within sight of the skyscrapers of San Francisco across the Bay. Somehow they came into contact with a substance to which Marsha was exceedingly sensitive. Within moments she showed symptoms of anaphylactic shock. They had gone off without a first-aid kit; however, Gretchen immediately did Therapeutic Touch. When Marsha had recovered, they walked back to camp, where they casually told us of the incident. Since then, there have been many such tales of emergency use of Therapeutic Touch, from babies being born in remote areas to older persons having heart attacks while living alone. "Happily," said Keith, a Therapeutic Touch therapist who had been able to help an elderly lady having a heart attack at a shopping mall, "I brought my hands along."

Teaching Therapeutic Touch to the Healee's Relatives

Because the basics of Therapeutic Touch are natural, safe, and easy to learn, for many years we have had a practice of teaching Therapeutic Touch to the relatives and friends of persons who are ill. This has been successful, and in many hospitals such programs have become accepted procedure—for instance, in hospital step-down units where relatives join in and learn the rehabilitation activities of patients awaiting discharge. It is also taught quite often to relatives accompanying patients receiving bone-marrow transplants at oncological centers; in pediatric units where parents have sleep-in arrangements; and other similar situations.

Peer Therapeutics in the Community

Another practice that has developed over the years we have named "peer therapeutics." Healees are often deeply touched by the efforts on their behalf during Therapeutic Touch sessions. Since Therapeutic Touch has such a high degree of safety, if they express an interest in doing Therapeutic Touch, we teach these healees the basic skills while they are in supervised settings. As they progress in Therapeutic Touch and their own health improves, we have them do it to persons who have the same illness that the former healee—now transposed to the role of healer—had. Perceiving the illness now from another perspective, the new Therapeutic Touch practitioner very often gains considerable insight into his or her own experiences as the healee. Often the insight has such a strong impact that it has been life-transforming.

In 1996, there are "peer therapeutic" groups active in several countries that are focused on health problems confronting persons with premenstrual syndrome; Raynaud's disease; cancers of many kinds; bilateral amputation; Graves' disease; AIDS; and postsilicon breast-implant symptoms; as well as among women's health groups, pregnant couples, and those with intrafamily problems. One of the most active groups formed is of members of the Gray Panthers, the political activist group of elderly persons, who do Therapeutic Touch to their same-age peers at nursing homes and senior retirement communities. However, one of the most thrilling—for its possible social consequences—has been an off-shoot of the "peer therapeutic" concept that was done first within the Oregon judicial system. In this program, teenaged delinquents who have been sentenced to periods of community service have been given the opportunity to learn Therapeutic Touch and then work off their time by doing it at facilities for the aged and the ill. It seems like a strange combination; however, apparently studies have demonstrated that grandparent figures can get closer to adolescents of our time than can parental figures, and perhaps Therapeutic Touch opens an opportunity for this relationship to happen.

Joining Therapeutic Touch with Other Therapies

Since we first introduced Therapeutic Touch a quarter-century ago, it has been taught to a broad spectrum of health professionals, beginning with nurses, doctors, and psychologists, and then spanning the whole array of licensed therapists, medical social workers, and counselors. One of the new fields in which Therapeutic Touch has been practiced concerns artificial insemination, and quite recently therapists who counsel persons adopting children have added Therapeutic Touch to their skills.

Therapeutic Touch has been found to interface well with all healing modalities, both traditional and orthodox, as well as more recent therapies, such as biofeedback. External Qi gong, the ancient Taoist art, has been called "The Chinese Therapeutic Touch" by one of its master teachers, Kenneth Cohen (Cohen, 1993). Persons who have combined massage with Therapeutic Touch practices have noted that although massage stimulates the client's energy field, it is Therapeutic Touch that truly balances it, and they recommend that Therapeutic Touch be part of all bodywork (Schatz and Carlson, 1995).

Therapeutic Touch and the "Other Nations"

In another instance, Therapeutic Touch has been used quite extensively with animals. A nun was one of the early "Krieger's Krazies," a term the first students of Therapeutic Touch coined for themselves and that has continued throughout the generations. After this nun completed her master's degree program in which Therapeutic Touch was part of the curriculum, she was granted a sabbatical for a year. She chose to spend the time herding sheep in the Rocky Mountains, and adapted Therapeutic Touch techniques during lambing time.

Shortly after the successful experience with the sheep, Therapeutic Touch began to be used with other farm animals. In several parts of the United States and Canada, it was found to be effective on horses and, later, cows. Very rapidly its use spread to goats, chickens, and ducks, and more recently, llamas. Now it is not unusual to find Therapeutic Touch being taught in a barn or out in the field, rather than in a formal classroom. However, that does not rule out classrooms: In one town in Vermont, persons learning Therapeutic Touch during a winter session brought their hens with them to practice on!

Therapeutic Touch on house pets has been in vogue since we first introduced it. Spotted here and there in communities across the country, clinics have been set up for the practice of Therapeutic Touch on cats, dogs, hamsters, white mice, and birds. They have been found to be unusually sensitive to Therapeutic Touch, the most remarkable aspect being the very rapid effect it has on birds.

Out of these developments has come a practice that may be the ultimate in compassionate regard for these "other nations." It was started by two stalwart "Krazies" in British Columbia, Janie and Liz, who taught Therapeutic Touch to a group of animal laboratory technicians. The lab technicians later used these skills on animals in their care before they were called upon to euthanize them. Such an act is without precedent, and I admit to not understanding my own mixed feelings about it. However, one message is clear to me: Never underestimate the power of compassion.

Worldwide Social Forces that Enabled Therapeutic Touch

Reviewing the history of Therapeutic Touch since its introduction, it is noticeable that its inception coincided with a remarkable window of time. More so than any other factor, this fortunate timing provided the right circumstances for the success of Therapeutic Touch. In a real sense, Dora Kunz and I were presented with an opportunity, and we accepted it.

Since World War II, there have been four social forces whose impact has reverberated to most countries throughout the world, and in doing so, they opened the way for the development of Therapeutic

Touch. Their energies have acted synergistically to produce unusual opportunities for significant changes in worldview, and this condition intensifies as the twenty-first century nears. In particular, this is a time of new beginnings. Carl Jung has called the 1990s an "End Point," because it is not only the end of a century, but also the end of a millennium. It is important, perhaps even crucial, that we now learn to think in new ways. It is time, Jung is saying, for a radical shift in perceptions. A significant transformation in the continuum of life is taking place as we flow into a new era and a new time, and we need to permit our fixed perceptions the latitude to perceive in new ways.

In the aftermath of World War II, both to escape the extensive devastations of the war, and to experience more fully the exotic and very different foreign cultures that came to light during the turmoil, *a worldwide urge to experience the new* took hold of people, and they traveled in hordes to the farthest reaches of the planet. On the dark side—coupled with voluntary travel during this time—there has been a period of mass migrations forced by the advances of natural catastrophes, such as drought, pestilence, and severe weather shifts which, sadly, have been attended by human frailities of avarice, cupidity, envy, and self-concern. However, the net result of these transnational migrations has been unparalleled; their interminglement of cultural mores on a grand scale has served to jolt many of this post-war generation into a realization of other cultural perspectives and an appreciation of other realities.

A second force that has significantly affected society has been *the post-war application of the many advances in science and technology* that were originally bred in the heat of warfare, but which were later adapted to the daily needs of people. Out of the understanding shaped by this high-tech upsurge that surrounds us in home, school, and the office, there arose a popular comprehension of the new physics behind the development of these modern utilities. The principles of relativity and quantum physics were sorted out for the common person and, as the concepts were translated into the "softer" sciences, the change in paradigm was felt very rapidly at the grass-roots. Crucial to this new frame of reference was a growing realization of the close correlation between the philosophy of the new science and the time-tested wisdom of ancient teachings, particularly those of the East.

A third force decisive in the acceptance of Therapeutic Touch—in fact, of all healing in our time—has been *the recognition of the power of the feminine principle in all people, regardless of gender.* This is a facet of human knowledge that has been lost to Western civilization, some think ever since biblical times. A major value of this acknowledgment has been an acceptance of the vulnerability that expression of compassion opens us to, and the recognition of it as an expression of strength rather than as a sign of weakness.

The fourth force that has aided the ground swell of acceptance of this permissive attitude has been *the reduced fear of death* that entered public consciousness under the compassionate prompting of Dr. Elisabeth Kubler-Ross. It was she who called forth in us the courage to recognize death as a part of life, encouraging us to make of life a meaningful event, and of death a celebration of that meaning.

There are many more social forces that were let loose in the second half of the twentieth century that created an atmosphere for the introduction of Therapeutic Touch and its acceptance, but I regard these four forces as crucial in sculpting an appropriate climate that made it easy and fun!

Simply stated they are:

- transcultural acceptance of other realities
- popular understanding of the philosophical implications of the new physics and realization of its close relationship to ancient teachings
- recognition of the significance of the feminine principle as a fundamental human characteristic
- reduction of the fear of death and a beginning acknowledgment that life has meaning.

One Significant Question Is Worth Many Answers

Looking back upon all of this, I continue to wonder at the question with which we began— *Why do I want to be healer?*—and realize that there is no one answer and that no answer is simple. Rather, answers grow in significance and in complexity as we begin to explore the depths and to realize the nature of the task we have put before ourselves. No sooner do we arrive at one level of understanding and seek to put the question to rest, than a slight shift in perspective opens another vista to be explored.

The process reminds me of a model for scientific inquiry that was posited to my class when I began my doctoral studies. We were gifted by having a remarkably brilliant, creative, and inspirational teacher, Professor Martha E. Rogers, who constantly encouraged us toward a goal of excellence. The model she put before us was Louis Agassiz, the renowned zoologist, geologist, and paleontologist of the nineteenth century, who was acknowledged to be far ahead of his time, both as a scientist and as a teacher.

The timeless story about him tells the tale of a young college student who aspired to be Agassiz's laboratory assistant. Arriving at the laboratory for his initial interview, the student was kept waiting several hours before Agassiz appeared. The room was bordered by specimens of fish of many kinds, and the student spent some of his waiting time studying the fish.

When Agassiz finally arrived and the brief introductory amenities were completed, the student made a polite remark about the array of fish. Agassiz asked him what he had noticed about the fish, and the student proudly reeled off an encyclopedic knowledge on the taxonomy of fish. After a while Agassiz said, "Yes, and what did you see?" The student was nonplussed, and only could stutter a poor reply. Agassiz said, "Yes, look again, look again," and he left. The student re-examined the fish until dark, when he went home.

He returned the next day. Agassiz was not around, and so the student went back to examining the fish. When Agassiz returned to the lab late in the day, the student read to him his litany of observations. With a nod of his head, Agassiz said," Yes. Look, look again!" and left.

Dark dreams of fish accompanied the student's troubled sleep that night. The next day he could hardly bring himself to face the task at hand, but he persisted. To his surprise he found features of the fish he had not noticed before. The new observations intrigued him, and he didn't notice Agassiz return. The story goes on a bit, but the bottom line is that the student finally finds the answer Agassiz is prodding him toward: The fish is symmetrical, and symmetry is the key to its successful survival as an aquatic being. Agassiz is pleased and the student gets the job but, as he is about to leave the room Agassiz turns, looks the student in the eye and encourages him on, firmly admonishing: "Look! Look again!"

It is with this charge, "Look, look again!" that I leave you. I have explored the question, *Why do I want to be healer?* for many years. To share with you the essence of my findings, I, too, would say: "Look! Look again!" The answer is in front of your eyes. Look again, and again.

APPENDIX A

Suggestions for Analyzing Your Inner Work Journal

Materials
Pen and paper, thesaurus, and a tape recorder.

Procedure
1. The prime practice that I have found most useful to an objective review of my journals is a negative: Do not read the journal for at least one to two weeks after writing it. When writing the journal, double space your entries and leave a two-inch margin along one side of the paper.
2. At the end of each two-week period, arrange a two-hour slot of time during which you will not be interrupted, and read that entire period's entries in one sitting. As you read and remember the events of the past two weeks, associated ideas, questions, insights, doodles, or sketches will come to mind. Jot them down in the margins of the paper and continue reading. At this time, also underline the key issues or ideas you have written about and words that stir an emotional reaction as you read your journal.
3. Go back over your journal, and in the empty lines (the double spaces) above the underlined words write their synonyms, which you can select from the thesaurus. You can add anything you wish in the margins at this time.
4. Reread your journal again; however, this time read it aloud into your tape recorder, substituting the synonyms for the original words.
5. Play back your tape recorder. As you listen, write down additional associated thoughts or comments in the margins of the paper.
6. Using your marginal notes as a guide, write a two to three paragraph summary of your current journal. Note areas you would like to follow up for further study or meditation.
7. Reread all of your summaries—or selected summaries—every three months. Evaluate how you have followed through on your ideas, questions, interests, and insights, and write up a broad plan to follow during the next three months.

APPENDIX B

Health Facilities Where Therapeutic Touch Is Practiced

Compiled by: Nurse Healers-Professional
Associates, Inc. Cooperative
(Listed alphabetically by state)

Hospice of the Valley
Dept: Home Care
2600 E. Thomas Road
Phoenix AZ 85016
Contact: Betty Croce
602-860-1995
Written Policy: No
Written Procedures: No

The Meadows
Dept: Addiction, recovery, psychiatry
PO Box 97
Wickenburg AZ 85358
Contact: Judy Lyn Sweetland, Staff RN
520-684-3926
520-684-3427
Melissa Gacke, RN, DON
Written Policy: Yes
Written Procedures: Yes
Taught Here: Yes

Alameda Hospital
Dept: Nursing
2070 Clinton Avenue
Alameda CA 94501
Contact: Christina Chapman, Staff Nurse III
510-814-4049
Written Policy: Yes
Written Procedures: Yes
Taught Here: Yes

Help Unlimited Home Care
1787 Goodyear
Ventura CA 93003
Contact: Marie Fasano-Ramos, RN
805-289-9999
Written Policy: Yes
Written Procedures: Yes
Taught Here: Yes

Hospice of Petaluma
Dept: Case Management
415 A Street
Petaluma CA 94952
Contact: Marilee Blonski, RN, Case
Manager
707-778-6242
Written Policy: Yes
Written Procedures: Yes
Taught Here: No

Mad River Hospital
3800 Janes Road
Arcata CA 95521
Contact: Stephanie Haines
707-677-3528 H
Written Policy: Yes
Written Procedures: Yes
Taught Here: Yes

Nursing Therapeutics Institute
170 East Cotati Avenue
Santa Rosa CA 94931
Contact: Phyllis Schubert, RN, DNSc, MA
707-795-1063
Rose Murray
Written Policy: Yes
Written Procedures: Yes
Taught Here: Yes

The New Radiance Holistic Health Nursing
Practice
PO Box 5142
San Mateo CA 94402
Contact: Chow Chow Imamoto, RN, MsD
415-341-1955
Written Policy: No
Written Procedures: No
Taught Here: Yes

Denver General Hospital
777 Bannock Street
Denver CO 80204

Contact: Marty Potter, Staff Development
303-839-5832

Written Policy: Yes
Written Procedures: Yes
Taught Here: Yes

Swedish Medical Center
501 East Hampden
Englewood CO 80110

Contact: Colleen Whalen, VP Clinical
  Services
303-788-5000

Written Policy: No
Written Procedures: No

Bristol Hospital
Brewster Road
Bristol CT 06010

Contact: Anne Minor, RN, TT Consultant
203-589-9984
Regina McNamara, VP, Patient Services
203-585-3041

Written Policy: Yes
Written Procedures: Yes
Taught Here: Yes

Griffin Hospital
Dept: Pastoral Care/Spirituality
Division Street
Derby CT 06418

Contact: Virginia Sheehan
413-734-8843

Written Policy: No
Written Procedures: No
Taught Here: Yes

Lawrence Memorial Hospital
Dept: OB
365 Montauk Avenue
New London CT 06320

Contact: Juanita Durham
203-444-5103
203-447-1111

Written Policy: No
Written Procedures: No (coming)

New Horizons Village
Dept: Health Services
37 Bliss Road
Unionville CT 06085

Contact: Marie Menut, Health Care
  Associate.
203-673-8893

Written Policy: No
Written Procedures: No
Taught Here: No

St. Vincent's Medical Center
Dept: DePaul Outpatient Psych Clinic
2800 Main Street
Bridgeport CT 06606

Contact: Barbara Krzyzer
203-576-5357
203-924-1758 H

Written Policy: No
Written Procedures: No

Chrysalis Natural Medicine Center
1008 Miltown Road
Wilmington DE 19808

Contact: Carolyn Murdic, Educational
  Coordinator
302-368-4340

Written Policy: Twice per year
Written Procedures: No

Bayfront Medical Center Community
  Resource Center
100 Second Avenue N Suite 100
St. Petersburg FL 33701

Contact: Shirley Spear-Begley
813-367-3063

Written Policy: No
Written Procedures: No
Taught Here: Every other month,
  2 days in length

Intro at Morton Plant Hospital, Training at
  Hospice of Florida Suncoast
Dept: Main Surgery
323 Jeffords Street
Clearwater FL 34617

Contact: Karen Murphy, Cardiac Clinician
813-462-7010

Written Policy: In process
Written Procedures: In process
Taught Here: Soon

Mercy Hospital
Dept: Infection Control
3663 S. Miami Avenue
Miami FL 33133

Contact: Barbara Terry
305-285-2706

Written Policy: Yes
Written Procedures: Yes
Taught Here: Yes

St. Anthony's Hospital
1200 7th Avenue North, PO Box 12588
St. Petersburg FL 33733

Contact: Shirley Spear-Begley
813-367-3063

Written Policy: No
Written Procedures: No
Taught Here: Every other month,
2 days in length

Boise State University
Dept: Nursing
1910 University Drive
Boise ID 83725-1840

Contact: Hilary Straub, Associate Professor
208-385-3782

Written Policy: No
Written Procedures: No
Taught Here: Yes

St. Francis Regional Medical Center
Dept: Surgical Intensive Care
929 N. St. Francis
Wichita KS

Contact: Barbara Denison, RN, BSN,
Staff RN
316-283-9146

Written Policy: No
Written Procedures: No
Taught Here: Yes

Murray-Calloway County Hospital
Dept: Staff Development
803 Poplar Street
Murray KY 42071

Contact: Kathy Culbert, RN, MSN, CS
502-762-1360
502-489-2284 H

Written Policy: No
Written Procedures: No
Taught Here: Yes

Ochsner Medical Foundation Hospital
1516 Jefferson Highway
New Orleans LA 70121

Contact: Regina Phelps, MN, RN, Nursing
Ed & Research
504-842-1891

Written Policy: Yes
Written Procedures: Yes
Taught Here: Yes

Our Lady of Lourdes Regional
Medical Center
611 St. Landry Street
Lafayette LA 70506

Contact: Darlene Lovas, RN, BSN, Nursing
Continuing Ed Specialist
318-289-2126

Written Policy: Pending
Written Procedures: Pending
Taught Here: Yes

Brigham's Women's Hospital
Dept: NICU, Nursing
75 Francis Street
Boston MA 02115

Contact: Steffanie Mulloney
508-470-1345
617-732-5420

Written Policy: No
Written Procedures: No

Heywood Hospital
Dept: Patient Care-Psychiatric Services
Mental Health Unit
242 Green Street
Gardner MA 01440

Contact: William Griffin, Director,
Psychiatric Services
508-630-6378

Written Policy: In process
Written Procedures: In process
Taught Here: Yes

Midcoast Hospital
Dept: Nursing
58 Baribeau Drive
Brunswick ME 04011

Contact: Karen Taber, Clinical Nurse
    Specialist
207-729-0181 ext 427
207-353-4875

Written Policy: Yes
Written Procedures: Yes
Taught Here: Yes

Craven Regional Medical Center
Dept: CVSICU
2000 Newse Blvd.
Atlantic Beach NC

Contact: Patti O'Rourke, Charge Nurse
919-633-8684

Written Policy: No
Written Procedures: No
Taught Here: Yes

Elliot Hospital
Dept: Pain Management
1 Elliot Way
Manchester NH 03103

Contact: Lorry Roy, Pain Clinic Manager
603-628-4486

Written Policy: No
Written Procedures: No
Taught Here: Yes

Odyssey House
Dept: Clinical
30 Winnacunnett Road
Hampton NH 03824

Contact: Linda A. Firth, RN
603-926-6702
508-462-1329

Written Policy: No
Written Procedures: No
Taught Here: Yes

PMS/ACT Women's Health Choices
Dept: Private Office
722 Route 3A
Bow NH 03106

Contact: Nyla Hiltz, RN, Owner
603-228-5650

Written Policy: No
Written Procedures: No
Taught Here: Yes

Southern New Hampshire Regional
    Medical Center
Dept: Nursing & Patient Care Services,
Med/Surg, ICU, NICU, Administration
PO Box 2014
Nashua NH 03060

Contact: Deborah Sampson
603-673-2258 H

Written Policy: Yes
Written Procedures: Yes

Christ Hospital
Dept: Home Health & Hospice
176 Palisade Avenue
Jersey City NJ 07306

Contact: Shelli Greenfield
201-762-1834

Classic Center for Health and Healing
25 Orchard Street Suite 101
Denville NJ 07834

Contact: Zoe Elva Putman, Director, MA,
    CMT
201-627-4833

Taught Here: Yes

Hospice Program of Hackensack Medical
    Center
Dept: Hospice
385 Prospect Avenue
Hackensack NJ 07010

Contact: Linda Gurick, RN, Hospice
    Director
201-342-7766
Mary Ann Collin, Director

Written Policy: Yes
Written Procedures: Yes

A & A Chiropractic
73-12 35 Avenue
Jackson Heights NY 11372-1738

Contact: Jonathan Lobl, Reflexologist
718-458-0616

Written Policy: No
Written Procedures: No
Taught Here: No

Albany Medical Center Hospital
Dept: Nursing Education
New Scotland Avenue
Albany NY
Contact: Connie Ogden, CRRN
212-271-6305
Written Policy: No
Written Procedures: No
Taught Here: Yes

Beth Israel Medical Center, NY
Dept: Nursing Education & Research,
  Nursing Administration
16th Street and 1st Avenue
New York NY 10003
Contact: Carolyn Drennan, RN, Supervisor
212-387-3923
Written Policy: No
Written Procedures: No
Taught Here: Yes

Columbia Presbyterian Medical Center
Dept: Nursing Education, and the Rosen-
  thal Center of Complementary Medicine
711 Fort Washington
New York NY 10032
Contact: Mary Kreider, MSN, TT
Workshop Coordinator
212-305-6635
Written Policy: No
Written Procedures: No
Taught Here: Yes

Community Nursing Organization
Dept: Visiting Nurse Service of New York
34-05 Steinway Street
Long Island City NY
Contact: Claire Durkin, Nurse Consultant
718-472-4848
718-347-7621
Written Policy: Pending
Written Procedures: Pending
Taught Here: Yes

MSKCC
Dept: Nursing Education
1275 York Avenue
New York NY 11209
Contact: Jo Rizzo, Clinical Instructor
212-639-7900 beeper #4168
Written Policy: No

Written Procedures: No
Taught Here: Yes

Parker Jewish Geriatric Institute
Dept: LTHHCP
5 Dakota Drive Suite 105
Lake Success NY 11042
Contact: Linda Hill
718-289-2700
718-289-2714
Written Policy: No
Written Procedures: No
Taught Here: Yes

Roswell Park Cancer Institute
Dept: Volunteer
Carlton and Elm Street
Buffalo NY 14263
Contact: Karen Vassh, RN
716-837-0129
Written Policy: Not yet
Written Procedures: Not yet
Taught Here: No

St. Mary's Hospital
Dept: Wellness Institute
427 Guy Park Avenue
Amsterdam NY 12010
Contact: Sr. Rita Jean Dubrey, Director
  of Wellness Institute
518-842-1900
Written Policy: Yes
Written Procedures: Yes
Taught Here: Yes

SUNY at Stony Brook
Dept: Family Health
Stony Brook NY 11794
Contact: Patricia Long, PhD, RN
Written Policy: No
Written Procedures: No
Taught Here: Yes

University Medical Center Stony Brook
Dept: throughout hospital/most services,
    Department of Psychiatry
University Medical Center
Stony Brook NY 11794

Contact: Carol Fairchild
516-444-1010
516-467-1392 H

Written Policy: No
Written Procedures: No

———

Visiting Nurse Service Home Care
Dept: Maternal Child Health
1250 Broadway 2nd Floor
New York NY 10117

Contact: Deirdra Kearney
212-889-8819

Written Policy: No
Written Procedures: No

———

Visiting Nurse Service Home Care in
    Manhattan
Dept: Education
1250 Broadway
New York NY 10117

Contact: Michelle Palamountain

Written Policy: No
Written Procedures: No
Taught Here: Yes

———

Visiting Nurse Service of New York
Dept: Hospice Care Program
1250 Broadway
New York NY 10001

Contact: Martha Fortune, Staff Nurse
212-290-3888

Written Policy: No
Written Procedures: No but charted
Taught Here: Yes

———

Winthrop-University Hospital
Dept: Nursing
259 First Street
Mineola NY 11501

Contact: Martha Baron, CNS
516-663-2780

Written Policy: Yes
Written Procedures: Yes
Taught Here: Yes

———

Mercy Hospital Anderson
Dept: Holistic Health & Wellness Center
7500 State Road
Cincinnati OH 45255

Contact: Anita Schambach, RN,
    Wellness Center
513-624-3232

Written Policy: Yes
Written Procedures: Yes
Taught Here: Yes

———

Metro Health Medical Center
Dept: Oncology
3395 Scranton Road
Cleveland OH 44109

Contact: Toni Kline
216-741-7988

Written Policy: No
Written Procedures: No

———

Riverside Methodist Hospital
Dept: Nursing
3535 Olentangy River Road
Columbus OH 43214

Contact: Marjorie Anderson, Clinical Nurse
    Specialist
614-566-5438

Written Policy: Yes
Written Procedures: Yes
Taught Here: Yes

———

Southwest General Health Center
Dept: Complementary Care Services
17951 Jefferson Park
Middleburg OH 44130

Contact: Marianne Montana, Director
216-816-6811

Written Policy: Not yet
Written Procedures: Not yet
Taught Here: Yes

———

Ashland Community Health Center
246 4th Street
Ashland OR 97520

Contact: Kelli LaFleur, RN, FNP
503-482-9741
503-482-4622 H

Written Policy: Yes
Written Procedures: Yes

Multnomah County Health Department
Dept: in the field
7944 SE 62nd Street
Portland OR 97206

Contact: Barbara Moore
503-774-5950

Written Policy: No
Written Procedures: No

Southern Oregon State College
Dept: Student Health Center
1250 Siskiyou
Ashland OR 97520

Contact: Susan Beardsley-Einhorn
503-488-5839

Written Policy: Yes
Written Procedures: Yes

Center for Human Integration
8400 Pine Road
Philadelphia PA 19111

Contact: Sheila McGinnis, Sr., Associate
   Director
215-742-8077

Written Policy: No
Written Procedures: No
Taught Here: Yes

Shadyside Hospital
Dept: Multidisciplinary Pain Program
5230 Centre Avenue
Pittsburgh PA 15232

Contact: Janet Ziegler
412-623-1201

Written Procedures: No

Choices for Healing
Dept: private practice
2934 Vaulx Lane
Nashville TN 37204

Contact: Bonnie Johnson, Nurse Healer,
   Owner

Written Policy: No
Written Procedures: No
Taught Here: Yes

Eastern State Hospital
4601 Ironbound Road
Williamsburg VA 23187

Contact: James Parham, Jr., RN, MA,
   Director of Staff Development

Written Policy: No
Written Procedures: No
Taught Here: Yes

Mt. Ascutney Hospital
Dept: Rehab
RR 1 Box 6 County Road
Windsor VT 05089

Contact: Carolyn Petell
802-674-4711 ext 292
Barbara Bruno
802-674-6711 ext 212

Written Policy: No
Written Procedures: No

Rutland Regional Medical Center
Dept: Oncology & throughout the hospital
160 Allen Street
Rutland VT 05701

Contact: Kit Morvan, Oncology Clinical
   Specialist
802-747-1693

Written Policy: No
Written Procedures: No
Taught Here: Yes

Southwestern Vermont Medical Center
Dept: Psychiatric Services
100 Hospital Drive East
Bennington VT 05201

Contact: Mimi Francis
802-447-5176
Ana Rosales

Written Policy: No
Written Procedures: Yes

Windham Center for Psychiatric Care
Dept: Psych-Mental Health
18 Old Terrace Court
Bellows Falls VT 05101

Contact: Stacey DeLuca
802-463-1346
802-824-6615 H

Written Policy: No
Written Procedures: No

Community Homewell Home Health
Dept: Nursing
1971 State Route 20
Sedro Wooley WA 98284

Contact: Rose Ann Dolan
206-376-6120

Written Policy: In process

Masonic Retirement Center
Dept: Nursing home, retirement for well
   elderly, frail elderly, health center
23660 Marine View Drive South
Des Moines WA 98198

Contact: Betty Green, ARNP
206-878-8980
Stacy Mesalos, Administrator

Written Policy: Yes
Written Procedures: Yes

Swedish Medical Center
Dept: Family Medicine
1101 Madison Suite 200
Seattle WA 98104

Contact: Kathi Kemper, MD
206-386-6228

Written Policy: No
Written Procedures: No

Virginia Mason Hospital and Clinic
Dept: Rehab Unit, Oncology
1100 9th, PO Box 900 c/o HNR9RHU
Seattle WA 98111

Contact: Sandra Revesz
206-624-1144 ext 4165
206-365-1127 H

Written Procedures: Yes

University of Wisconsin Milwaukee,
   Silver Spring
Dept: Community Nursing Center
5460 North 64th Street
Milwaukee WI 53218

Contact: Bev Zabler, RN, RNP
414-463-7950
414-534-4621

Taught Here: Yes

Foothills Hospital
Dept: Out-patient & some in-patient taught
   to students of nursing
1403 29th Street NW
Calgary AB T2N 2T9

CANADA
Contact: Linda Terra
403-238-3734
Marney Armitage
403-242-3549

Written Policy: No
Written Procedures: No

Mayfair Nursing Home
Dept: Nursing Home
8240 Collicut Street SW
Calgary AB T2V 2X1
CANADA

Contact: Linda Terra
403-238-3734

Written Policy: No
Written Procedures: No
Taught Here: No

Rockyview Hospital
Dept: Out-patient & some in-patient taught
   to students of nursing
707 14th Street SW
Calgary AB T2V 1P9
CANADA

Contact: Marney Armitage
403-242-3549

Written Policy: No
Written Procedures: No
Taught Here: Yes

Royal Alexander Hospital
Dept: Emergency Room
10240 Kingsway Avenue
Edmonton AB P5H 3V9
CANADA

Contact: Maureen Dundin
403-476-8860

Written Policy: No
Written Procedures: No

Tom Baker Cancer Centre
Dept: Out-patient & some in-patient taught
   to students of nursing
1331 29th Street NW
Calgary AB T2N 4N2
CANADA

Contact: Marney Armitage
403-242-3549

Written Policy: No
Written Procedures: No

Calgary General Hospital, Bow Valley
  Centre
841 Centre Avenue East
Calgary AB T2E 0A1
CANADA
Contact: Linda Terra
403-238-3734
Diana Law, Director of Nursing
Written Policy: Yes
Written Procedures: Yes
Taught Here: Yes

B.C. Cancer Agency, Vancouver Clinic
Dept: Patient & Family Counseling
600 West 10th Avenue
Vancouver BC V5Z 4E6
CANADA
Contact: Sarah Sample
604-877-6000 ext 2194
Lis Smith, Clinical Hypnotherapist
604-877-6000 ext 2188
Written Policy: In process
Written Procedures: In process

B.C. Cancer Agency, Vancouver Island
Dept: Patient & Family Counseling
1900 Fort Street
Victoria BC V8R 1J8
CANADA
Contact: Michael Boyle
604-595-9230
Written Policy: Yes
Written Procedures: No

Capital Region District Health Clinic Office
Dept: Community Health
1947 Cook Street
Victoria BC V8T 3P8
CANADA
Contact: Kathy Gilchrist
604-595-3284
Victoria General Hospital (GFHS), Labor
  and Delivery
Nora Walker
604-388-4562
35 Helmicken Road
Victoria BC V8Z 6R5 CANADA
Written Policy: No
Written Procedures: No

Fraser Burrard Hospital Society, Royal
  Columbian Site

Dept: Nursing, Staffing
530 Columbia Street
New Westminster BC V3L 3W7
CANADA
Contact: Joanne Carol Nielson
604-943-2816
Written Policy: Yes
Written Procedures: Yes

Lady Minto Hospital
Dept: Extended Care
Box 307
Ganges BC V0S 1E0
CANADA
Contact: Carol Spencer
604-537-5545
Written Policy: In progress
Written Procedures: In progress

Langley Mental Health Centre
Dept: Child & Youth Services
2300 Fraser Highway Suite 305
Langley BC Z3A 4E6
CANADA
Contact: Anna Fritz
604-532-3500
604-737-1098
Written Policy: No
Written Procedures: No

St. Paul's Hospital
Dept: Nursing, Room 404 Burrand
1081 Burrand Street
Vancouver BC V6Z 1Y6
CANADA
Contact: Mark Turris, RN
604-986-2732
Theresa Thompson, CNS
604-682-2344
Written Policy: Yes
Written Procedures: Yes

Tofino General Hospital
Dept: General Care
Tofino BC V0R 2Z0
CANADA
Contact: Priscilla Lockwood
604-725-3303
Written Policy: No
Written Procedures: No

UAN Public Health Department
Dept: Home Care
1060 West 8th Avenue
Vancouver BC V6H 1C4
CANADA

Contact: Lynette Morrison
604-261-6366

Written Policy: Yes
Taught Here: No

Victoria General Hospital
Dept: throughout hospital
2819 Inlet Avenue
Victoria BC V9A 2M6
CANADA

Contact: Jeannette Merryfield
604-383-5517

Written Policy: In progress
Written Procedures: In progress

University of New Brunswick
Dept: Extensions & Continuing Education:
   Faculty of Nursing
PO Box 4400
Fredericton NB E3B 5A3
CANADA

Contact: Barbara Cull-Wilby, Professor
506-453-4642
L. Ouellette, Professor

Written Policy: No
Written Procedures: No

Etobicoke General Hospital
Dept: ICU PACU
101 Humber College Boulevard
Etobicoke ON
CANADA

Contact: Mary Bant, RN
416-747-3313
Lidia Tucker, RN
416-747-3558

Taught Here: No

Guelph Wellington Duff (VON)
   Community Nursing
Dept: Nursing
RR 4
Orangeville ON L9W 2Z1
CANADA

Contact: Jane Richmond
519-941-3100

Written Policy: Yes
Written Procedures: Yes

Pembroke Civic Hospital
425 Cecelia Street
Pembroke ON K8A 1S7
CANADA

Contact: Sheila Watt, RN
613-735-4706

Written Policy: Yes
Written Procedures: Yes

St. Joseph's Health Center
30 The Queen's Way
Toronto ON M6R 1B5
CANADA

Contact: Margaret Blastorah, Clinical
   Nursing Coordinator
416-534-9531

Written Policy: Yes
Written Procedures: Yes
Taught Here: Yes

Toronto East General Hospital and
   Orthopedic Hospital
Dept: Nursing
825 Coxwell Avenue
Toronto ON M4C 3E7
CANADA

Contact: Shirley Dalglish, RN, Coordinator
   Palliative Care
416-469-6431
43 Pitcairn Crescent
Toronto ON M4A 1P5
CANADA

Written Policy: Yes
Written Procedures: Yes
Taught Here: Yes

Victoria Hospital Corporation
Dept: ICU
375 South Street
London ON N6A 4G5
CANADA

Contact: Myra Apostle-Mitchell
519-453-7041
519-473-1165

Written Policy: In process
Written Procedures: In process

Victoria Order of Nurses, Peel Branch
Dept: VON Community Nursing
1760 Argentia Street Unit 3
Mississauga ON L5N 3A9
CANADA

Contact: Nancy Hall
905-793-5476

Written Policy: In process
Written Procedures: In process

Victorian Order of Nurses (VON) Simcoe
   County Branch
Dept: Alzheimer Respite Program
54 Cedar Pointe Drive   Unit 1207
Barrie ON L4N 5R7
CANADA

Contact: Evy Cugelman
705-737-4990

Written Policy: Yes
Written Procedures: Yes

Cope Foundation
Dept: Physical Therapy, Nursing Units,
   Special School
Bonnington, Montenotte, Cork
IRELAND

Contact: Leonie Smith
353-021-871559

Written Policy: No
Written Procedures: No

Nursing Midwifery and Health Department:
Christchurch Polytechnic
PO Box 22-095
Christchurch
NEW ZEALAND

Contact: Jean Beynon, Education
033-798150

Taught Here: To be integrated

Holy Family Hospital
Dept: Primary Health Care
PO Box 21
Berekum BA Ghana
WEST AFRICA

Contact: Sr. Margaret Moran, PHC
   Fieldworker
215-742-6100

Written Policy: No
Written Procedures: No
Taught Here: Soon

APPENDIX C

Schools Where Therapeutic Touch is Taught

Compiled by: Nurse Healers-Professional
Associates, Inc. Cooperative
(Listed alphabetically by state)

University of Alabama at Birmingham,
UAV Station
Dept: School of Nursing
1701 University Blvd. Room GO10
Birmingham AL 35294

Contact: Ann Clark, Doctor
205-934-6639

Taught as Part of Curriculum? Graduate
school elective
Frequency Taught: Weekly for 3 hours

Arizona State University
Dept: College of Nursing
Tempe AZ 85287-2602

Contact: Katherine Matas, RN, PhD
602-965-4918

Taught as Part of Curriculum? Continuing
education and elective course
Frequency Taught: 2 times per year

California State University at Long Beach
Dept: Nursing
1350 Bellflower Blvd.
Long Beach CA 90840

Contact: Nancy Oliver, RN, PhD

Taught as Part of Curriculum? Independent
study-graduate
Frequency Taught: Every semester-spring/
fall

Chaffey College
Dept: Physical Education/Wellness Division
5885 Haven Avenue
Rancho CA 91701-0430

Contact: Marilyn Shaw, Professor
909-941-2324

Taught as Part of Curriculum? Elective
Frequency Taught: 1 time per year

College of the Redwoods
Dept: Nursing
Tompkins Hill Road
Eureka CA 95503

Contact: Janne Gibbs
707-445-6873
707-443-2697

Taught as Part of Curriculum? Yes
Frequency Taught: Integrated in clinical

Frontiers in Nursing Education
435 Rose Avenue
Mill Valley CA 94941

Contact: Sharon Kane, RN
415-383-5076

Frequency Taught: 2-4 times per year

Hospice Services of Lake County
PO Box 1430
Clearlake CA 95422-1430

Contact: Kathy Fielding, Director of
Professional Services
707-994-8820

Sacramento City College
Dept: Associate Degree Nursing,
Continuing Education
3835 Freeport Blvd.
Sacramento CA 95822-1386

Contact: Rae Wood, Nursing Instructor
916-449-7271
Marie Jenkins, Nursing Instructor
916-687-6923

Taught as Part of Curriculum? No
Frequency Taught: 3 times per year

San Francisco State University
Dept: Institute for Holistic Studies
1600 Holloway Avenue
San Francisco CA 94132

Contact: Erik Peper
415-338-1210

Taught as Part of Curriculum? Elective-part
of continuing education
Frequency Taught: 1 time per year

———————————————————

Metropolitan State College of Denver
Dept: NUR and HCN Campus Box 33
PO Box 173 362
Denver CO 80217-3362

Contact: DC Kathleen McGuire Mahony,
Chair
303-556-3130

Taught as Part of Curriculum? Yes
Frequency Taught: 1 time

———————————————————

Red Rocks Community College
Dept: Nursing Continuing Education
3300 West 6th Avenue, Box 27
Lakewood CO 80401-5398

Contact: Carol Baden, Dept. Chair, Health
Occupations
303-988-6160

Frequency Taught: 2 times per semester for
3 semesters

———————————————————

University of Colorado
Dept: School of Nursing
4200 East 9th Avenue Campus Box C288
Denver CO 80262

Contact: Janet Quinn
303-270-5592
303-449-5790 H

Taught as Part of Curriculum? Elective
Frequency Taught: 1 time per year

———————————————————

Howard University College of Nursing
Dept: Nursing
Bryant Street
Washington DC

Contact: Shirley Robinson, Assistant
Professor
202-806-3753

Frequency Taught: Every semester

———————————————————

Georgetown University
Dept: School of Nursing
3700 Reservoir Road NW
Washington DC 20007

Contact: Judith Baigis-Smith, Associate Dean
301-365-1906 H
Irene Morelli
202-687-5127

Taught as Part of Curriculum? Integrated
into nursing courses
Frequency Taught: Spring

———————————————————

Educating Hands School of Massage
Therapy
261 West 8th Street
Miami FL 33130

Contact: Karen Fransbergen
1-800-999-6991

Taught as Part of Curriculum? No
Frequency Taught: Sporadic

———————————————————

Santa Fe Community College
Dept: Associate of Science in Nursing
3000 NW 83rd Street
Gainesville FL 32606

Contact: Pat Simmons
904-395-5750

Taught as Part of Curriculum? Yes
Frequency Taught: Each class

———————————————————

St. Petersburg Junior College
Dept: Nursing Health Education
7200 66th Street
N. Pinellas Park FL 33709

Contact: Jody Parks, Dean of College of
Nursing
813-341-3618
Shirley Spear-Begley
813-367-3063

Taught as Part of Curriculum? No
Frequency Taught: Sporadic

———————————————————

The Humanities Center (School of Massage)
4045 Park Blvd.
Pinellas Park FL 34665

Contact: Sherry Fears, Director of Education
813-541-5200

Taught as Part of Curriculum? No
Frequency Taught: 2-3 times per year

———————————————————

University of Central Florida
Dept: Nursing
1519 Clearlake Road
Cocoa FL 32922

Contact: Patricia Stanley, Instructor
407-632-1111 ext. 65571

Taught as Part of Curriculum? No
Frequency Taught: 2-3 times per year

University of South Florida
Dept: College of Nursing
12901 Bruce B. Downs Blvd. Box 22
Tampa FL 33612-4799

Contact: Joyce Larson
813-974-9119
Shirley Spear-Begley
813-367-3063

Taught as Part of Curriculum? No
Frequency Taught: 1 time per semester

University of Hawaii at Manoa
Dept: College of Continuing Education &
    Community Service
2530 Dole Street
Honolulu HI 96822

Contact: Carol Trockman
808-528-1157

Taught as Part of Curriculum? No
Frequency Taught: once per semester

The Alverno Health Care Facility
Dept: Nursing
849 13th Avenue North
Clinton IA 52732

Contact: Phyllis Doe, DON
319-242-1521

Taught as Part of Curriculum? Is to be part
of orientation

Idaho State University
Dept: Nursing
Box 8101
Pocatello ID 83209

Contact: Grace Jacobson, Assistant
Professor
208-236-2437

Taught as Part of Curriculum? Yes
Frequency Taught: 1 semester

Lewis-Clark State College
Dept: Nursing
500 8th Avenue
Lewiston ID 83501

Contact: Susie Bunt, Associate Professor
208-734-2443

Taught as Part of Curriculum? No, as an
elective
Frequency Taught: Every other year or on
demand

College of Dupage
Dept: Nursing
22nd and Lambert Road
Glen Ellyn IL 60137

Contact: Mary Gayle Floden, Professor
of Nursing
708-858-2800 ext. 2536

Taught as Part of Curriculum? Yes in
nursing
Frequency Taught: Every quarter

St. Xavier University
Dept: School of Nursing
3700 West 103rd Street
Chicago IL 60655

Contact: Joan M. Hau, Assistant Dean,
Graduate Nursing
312-298-3708

Taught as Part of Curriculum?
Informally only
Frequency Taught: Varies

Indiana University/Kokomo
Dept: Nursing
2300 S. Washington
Kokomo IN 46904

Contact: Judy Lausch
317-455-9264

Taught as Part of Curriculum? Elective only
Frequency Taught: Each semester

Valparaiso University
Dept: School of Nursing
Valparaiso IN 46383

Contact: Barbara Starke, Adjunct Assistant
616-849-1239

Taught as Part of Curriculum? Optional
Frequency Taught: 1 semester

Cloud County Community Hospital
Dept: Nursing
PO Box 507
Beloit KS 67420
Contact: Gayle Sewell
913-738-2259
913-738-5045 H

School of Nursing Wichita State University
Dept: School of Nursing
Box 41 Ahlberg Hall
Wichita KS 67208
Contact: Diana Guthrie, Professor
316-261-2631
Taught as Part of Curriculum? Fall 95
Frequency Taught: New class

Wesley Medical Center
Dept: Education
550 North Hillside
Wichita KS 67214
Contact: Bee Vrzak
Taught as Part of Curriculum? No
Frequency Taught: 1-2 times per year

Murray State University
Dept: Nursing
PO Box 9
Murray KY 42071
Contact: Nancey France, Director
502-762-2193
Taught as Part of Curriculum? Elective
Frequency Taught: Annual

Total Health, Inc. - Associates in Holistic
  Nursing
Dept: Continuing Education
650 Teddy Street
Slidell LA 70458
Contact: Mary Frost, CE Instructor
504-893-3890
504-641-2418
Julie Nelson, CE Instructor
504-641-2418
Frequency Taught: Several times per year

Simmons College School for Health Studies
Dept: Graduate Nursing
300 The Fenway
Boston MA 02215-5898
Contact: Carol Wells-Federman, RN

617-632-7374
Steffanie Mulloney
508-470-1345
Taught as Part of Curriculum? Yes
Frequency Taught: Annually

University of Massachusetts/Amherst
Dept: School of Nursing
325 Arnold House, University of
  Massachusetts
Amherst MA 01003
Contact: Mary Ann Bright, RN, LS, EdD
413-545-1344
413-253-5855
Taught as Part of Curriculum? Elective
Frequency Taught: Sporadic

UMAB School of Nursing
Dept: Acute & Long Term Care
622 St. Lombard Street
Balto MD 21201
Contact: Margaret McEntee, RN, PhD
410-706-3847
Taught as Part of Curriculum? Yes
Frequency Taught: Spring and summer
  semester

University of Southern Maine
Dept: School of Nursing
96 Falmouth Street
Portland ME 04103
Contact: Dorothy Woods Smith, PhD, RN,
  Associate Professor
207-780-4797
Jane Comman, Assistant Professor
207-780-4404
Taught as Part of Curriculum? Elective
Frequency Taught: 2 times per year

Delta College
Dept: Adult/Community Education
University Center
Saginaw MI 48710
Contact: Mary Ann Jordan
517-792-9380 H
Taught as Part of Curriculum? No
Frequency Taught: Each month

Holistic Health Center
29200 Vassar #140
Livonia MI 48152

Contact: Kathy Sinnett, Director
810-471-7010

Taught as Part of Curriculum? No
Frequency Taught: Each month

Michigan State University
Dept: College of Nursing
A230 Life Sciences
East Lansing MI 48912

Contact: Sharon Dimmer, Professor
517-484-5215
Gwen Wyatt, Associate Professor
517-353-6672

Taught as Part of Curriculum? Elective
Frequency Taught: 491 fall semester,
    591 spring semester

University of Minnesota
Dept: School of Nursing
6401 HSUF 308 Harvard SE
Minneapolis MN 55455

Contact: Ellen Egan, Associate Program
612-624-1141

Taught as Part of Curriculum? Elective
Frequency Taught: 1 day per week every
    other year

St. Joseph Hospital
Dept: Taught by TT networkers group with
    permission of hospital
Kinsley Street
Nashua NH 03060

Contact: Norma Barnett, RN
603-673-5997

Frequency Taught: 3 times per year

Jersey City State College
Dept: Nursing
2039 Kennedy Blvd.
Jersey City NJ 07305

Contact: Barbara Collett, Professor
201-200-3264

Taught as Part of Curriculum? Yes, as a
nursing elective
Frequency Taught: Each semester

Ocean County College
Dept: The Center for Nursing and Allied
    Health Continuing Education

Colley Drive PO Box 2001
Ioms River NJ 08754-2001

Contact: Carol Gurdjian, RN, BSN
908-255-0404

Frequency Taught: 1 time per year

Our Lady of Lourdes Wellness Center
900 Haddon Avenue
Collingswood NJ 08108

Contact: Sheila McGinnis
215-742-8077

Frequency Taught: 1 time per year

Salem Community Collge
Dept: Nursing
560 Hollywood Avenue
Carney's Point NJ 08069

Contact: Louise Murphy, Director of
    Nursing
609-351-2648

Taught as Part of Curriculum?
    Fundamentals of nursing
Frequency Taught: Integrated throughout
    curriculum

Somerset School Massage Therapy
7 Cedar Grove Lane
Somerset NJ 08873

Contact: Susen Edwards, Owner, Instructor
908-356-0787

Taught as Part of Curriculum? No
Frequency Taught: 2-4 times per year

Binghamton University
Dept: Decker School of Nursing #4
PO Box 6000 Binghamton University
Binghamton NY 13902-6000

Contact: Jo Straneva, Assistant Professor
607-777-6704

Taught as Part of Curriculum? Yes
Frequency Taught: 3 times per year

College of New Rochelle
Dept: Graduate Nursing
29 Castle Place
New Rochelle NY 10804

Contact: Ellen McMahon
914-337-7300 ext. 4991
914-235-2315 H

Taught as Part of Curriculum? Yes

Hunter College/City University of
New York
Dept: Hunter-Bellevue School of Nursing
525 East 25th Street
New York NY 10010

Contact: Violet Malinski, PhD, RN
212-481-5102
914-779-5850 H

Taught as Part of Curriculum? Elective
Frequency Taught: Approximately every
18 months

Molloy College
Dept: Continuing Education
1000 Hempstead Avenue
Rockville Centre NY 11570

Contact: Marion Lowenthal, Coordinator
516-678-5000

Taught as Part of Curriculum? No
Frequency Taught: 1-2 times per semester

Orange County Community College
Dept: Non-Credit Continued Education
115 South Street
Middletown NY 10940

Contact: Antoinette Sardella
914-343-0640

Taught as Part of Curriculum? No

Pace University School of Nursing
Dept: Graduate Nursing
Redford Road
Pleasantville NY 10520

Contact: Patricia Blagman
914-773-3555

Taught as Part of Curriculum? Graduate
elective
Frequency Taught: Every spring semester

Capital University School of Nursing &
Adult Degree Program
Dept: ADP/BSN
2199 East Main Street
Columbus OH 43209

Contact: Kate Dean-Haidet, MSN, RNCS
614-236-6703

Taught as Part of Curriculum? Yes
Frequency Taught: 2 times per year

Cleveland State University
Dept: Continuing Education
East 24th and Euclid Avenue
Cleveland OH 44115

Contact: Linda Durham
216-295-0673
Toni Kline
216-749-3763

Taught as Part of Curriculum? CE
Frequency Taught: 2 times per year

Franklin University
Dept: School of Nursing
201 South Grant Avenue
Columbus OH 43215

Contact: Marjorie Anderson, Clinical
Nurse Specialist
614-566-5438

Taught as Part of Curriculum? Yes, special
topics course, optional
Frequency Taught: 1 time per year

Hocking College
Dept: School of Nursing
3301 Hocking Way
Nelsonville OH 45764

Contact: Suselma Roth, MSN, RN
614-753-3591

Taught as Part of Curriculum? Health
promotion elective

Kent State University
Dept: School of Nursing
Henderson Hall
Kent OH 44242

Contact: Sherron Herdtner, Assistant
Professor
216-672-3686
216-673-0594

Taught as Part of Curriculum? No-
continuing education
Frequency Taught: Yearly

Mount Carmel College of Nursing
127 South Davis Avenue
Columbus OH 43222

Contact: Kathy Lennon
614-263-6557 H

Taught as Part of Curriculum? Yes-
elective nursing seminar

Oregon Health Science University
Dept: School of Nursing at Southern
   Oregon State College
1250 Siskiyou
Ashland OR 97520

Contact: Susan Beardsley-Einhorn
503-488-5839

Taught as Part of Curriculum? Yes-elective,
   2 credits, graded
Frequency Taught: 1 time every 2 years

Center for Human Integration
8400 Pine Road
Philadelphia PA 19111

Contact: Sheila McGinnis, Sr., Associate
   Director
215-742-8077

Taught as Part of Curriculum? No
Frequency Taught: In 2 parts-1 time
   per semester

University of Rhode Island
Dept: Nursing/Health Services
White Hall/URI
Kingston RI 02881

Contact: Denise Cooper, RN
401-792-2766

Taught as Part of Curriculum? No
Frequency Taught: 1 time per semester

UTMB-SON
1100 Mechanic
Graineston TX 77550

Contact: Machele Clark, Associate
Professor
409-772-1237
Marsha Ford

Taught as Part of Curriculum? Yes, for
   elective
Frequency Taught: 1-2 times per year

College of Health Sciences
PO Box 13186
Roanoke VA 24031

Contact: Mary Jane Witter, MS, RN
703-985-8483

Taught as Part of Curriculum? No
Frequency Taught: Sporadic, 3 times in past

H.J. Reilly School of Massotherapy
67th Street and Atlantic Avenue
Virginia Beach VA 23451

Contact: Elaine Hruska, Instructor
804-428-0446

Taught as Part of Curriculum? Yes
Frequency Taught: 2 times per year
   (for each massage class)

Riverside School of Professional Nursing
500 J. Clyde Morris Blvd.
Newport News VA 23601

Contact: Maryann Ford, Director
804-594-2714

Taught as Part of Curriculum? Yes
Frequency Taught: Since 95

Virginia School of Massage
Charlottesville VA

Contact: Sue Ellus Dyer, Administrator
804-293-4031

Frequency Taught: 1-2 times per year

Castleton State College
Dept: Nursing
Castleton VT

Contact: Kit Morvan
802-747-1693

Taught as Part of Curriculum? No
Frequency Taught: 1 time per semester

Norwich University
Dept: School of Nursing
Montpelier VT 05602

Contact: Kit Morvan
802-747-1693

Taught as Part of Curriculum? Yes
Frequency Taught: 2 times per year

Alexander's School of Natural Therapeutics
4032 Pacific Avenue
Tacoma WA 98408

Contact: Aleisha Alexander
206-473-1142
206-365-1127 H
Sandy Revesz

Taught as Part of Curriculum? Yes
Frequency Taught: 4 times per year

Highline Community College
Dept: Nursing
23660 Marine Club Drive South
Des Moines WA 98198

Contact: Betty Green
206-878-8980 ext. 8434

Taught as Part of Curriculum? Extra
Frequency Taught: 2 times per year

Intercollegiate Center for Nursing
    Education Washington State University
Dept: Nursing
421 South 28 Avenue
Yakima WA 98902

Contact: Pat Aarmodt, Faculty &
    Coordinator
509-575-2130

Taught as Part of Curriculum? Yes
Frequency Taught: Each semester

Virginia Mason Medical Center
Dept: Nursing Education
1100 9th Avenue PO Box 900 c/o
    HNR9RHU
Seattle WA 98111

Contact: Sandra Revesz c/o Rehab Unit,
    9th Floor
206-624-1144 ext. 4165

Taught as Part of Curriculum? Continuing
    education
Frequency Taught: 1 time per year

University of Wisconsin/Milwaukee
Dept: School of Nursing-Continuing
    Education & Outreach
UW-Milwaukee, PO Box 4141
Milwaukee WI 53201

Contact: Bev Zabler, MS, RN, FNP
414-463-7950
414-534-4621

Taught as Part of Curriculum? Continuing
    education
Frequency Taught: 1-2 times per year

Viterbo College
Dept: School of Nursing
815 9th Street
LaCrosse WI 54601

Contact: Joan Keller Maresh,
    Associate Professor
608-791-0205

Taught as Part of Curriculum? As part of a
    nursing course
Frequency Taught: Annually

The Flinders University
Dept: School of Nursing-Faculty of Health
    Science
PO Box 2100
Adelaide South 5051
SOUTH AUSTRALIA

Contact: Lesley Cuthbertson, MS
08-201-3494

Frequency Taught: 1-2 times per year

Flinders University of South Australia
Dept: Faculty of Health Sciences/School of
    Nursing
Sturt Road
Bedford Park SA 5042
AUSTRALIA

Contact: Amy Bartjes, Senior Lecturer
08-201-33-12

Taught as Part of Curriculum? Yes
Frequency Taught: 1-2 times per year

University of Alberta
Dept: Faculty of Extension
University Extension Center, 93 University
    Campus NW
Edmonton AB T6G 2T4
CANADA

Contact: Merle Martin
403-434-3858

Taught as Part of Curriculum? Extension
    course
Frequency Taught: 4 times per year

Edmonton Public Schools/Edmonton
    General Hospital
Dept: Daily Living & Human Interest
    Course
1111 Jasper Avenue
Edmonton AB T6C 2C1
CANADA

Contact: Rhonda Ashmore, Program
    Manager
403-479-1104

Frequency Taught: As requested

The Center College for Wholistic Studies
10991-124 Street
Edmonton AB T5M 0H9
CANADA
Contact: Shelley Winton, RN
403-454-3279
Frequency Taught: 1-2 times per term

Mid-Island Health Education Society
513 Westview Place
Nanaimo BC V9V 1B3
CANADA
Contact: Phyllis Coleman, RN
Taught as Part of Curriculum? Optional
Frequency Taught: Varies

University of Victoria
Dept: School of Nursing
PO Box 1700 MS 7955
Victoria BC V8W 2Y2
CANADA
Contact: Barbara Courtney-Young, RN,
    BSN, Program Coordinator of
    Continuing Education
Taught as Part of Curriculum? No

Georgian College
Dept: School of Continuous Learning
1 Georgian Drive
Barrie ON L4M 3X9
CANADA
Contact: Evy Cugelman
705-737-4990
705-734-0412 H
Taught as Part of Curriculum? No
Frequency Taught: 3-4 times per year

Loyalist College
Dept: Night School-Continuing Education
PO Box 4200
Belleville ON L4M 3X9
CANADA
Contact: Donna Logan VanVleit
613-962-1004
Taught as Part of Curriculum? Continuing
    education
Frequency Taught: 3 times per year

Peel Memorial Hospital
Dept: Birthing Centre
20 Lunch Street

Brampton ON L6W 2Z6
CANADA
Contact: Mary Simpson, Instructor
905-454-2688
Frequency Taught: In progress

Sault College
Dept: Continuing Education (Nursing)
Box 60
Sault St. Marie ON P6A 5L3
CANADA
Contact: Bert Simpson
905-759-2554
Taught as Part of Curriculum? No
Frequency Taught: 2 times per year

University of Toronto
Dept: Faculty of Nursing
50 St. George Street
Toronto ON M5S 1A1
CANADA
Contact: Diane May
905-897-8761
Penny Birrell
Taught as Part of Curriculum? Yes
Frequency Taught: Semi-annually

University of Western Ontario
Dept: Faculty of Part-Time & Continuing
    Education
Room 23, Stevenson-Ianson Building
London ON N6A 5B8
CANADA
Contact: Sara Steems, Director
519-661-3631
Taught as Part of Curriculum? Continuing
    education
Frequency Taught: Oct-Nov, Feb-Mar,
    April-May

Cope Foundation
Dept: In- Service Education: Nurses/
    Teachers/Assistants/Psychologists
Bonnington
Montenotte Cork Eire
IRELAND
Contact: Leonie Smith
353-021-507131
Taught as Part of Curriculum? No
Frequency Taught: 1 time per term

GLOSSARY

AUTONOMIC NERVOUS SYSTEM: A part of the nervous system which is concerned with reflex control of bodily functions, such as the glands, smooth muscle tissue, and the heart.

CENTERING: Focusing the consciousness in the heart region and experiencing that state in an act of interior quietude.

CHAKRA: Supraphysical center of consciouness.

CHEMICAL BONDS: Force holding atoms together in a molecule or crystal.

CUES: Subjective signals perceived by the therapist during the Therapeutic Touch assessment of the energy fields of the healee's personal self.

FIELD: A region in which a force is effective; the force is exerted in such an area; a hypothetical "condition" produced in space. For example, in relation to the human personal self:

1. Conceptual field: Supraphysical unitive foundation of all avenues of consciousness of the personal self. Interpenetrates the pschodynamic field, the vital-energy field, and the physical body.

2. Psychodynamic field: Supraphysical domain of the emotions of the personal self. Interpenetrates the vital-energy field and the physical body.

3. Vital-energy field: Supraphysical energy state that interpenetrates and vitalizes the physical body.

HEMIPLEGIS: Paralysis of one side of the body.

HOLOGRAM: A three-dimensional image formed by the interference of light beams from a coherent light source; a photograph of the interference pattern which when suitably illuminated produces a three-dimensional image.

HUMAN ENERGY FIELD: Complex of several interpenetrating energy fields of the personal self (see above), which includes the electromagnetic field, the gravitational field, and weak and strong nuclear forces.

INTENTIONALITY: Purposive behavior.

KANDA: Supraphysical site in the root chakra (*muladhara*, Skt.) from which the nadis arise.

KUNDALINI: Creative force seated in a latent form within the root chakra.

LILA: Sport or amusement.

MANTRA: The root "man" (Skt.) means to think; an instrument of thought; a power in the form of sound.

METANEEDS: Human needs of a high order or imperative that are beyond those required for survival.

NADIS: Supraphysical energy circuits.

NEUROPEPTIDES: Messenger molecules made up of amino acids; can cause alterations of mood, pain, and pleasure.

OPEN ENERGY SYSTEM: In reference to human beings, an organized body of bioenergies that stream in continual flow into, through, and out of the biological systems.

ORDER: Gives meaning to events happening in space and time. For example (re. David Bohm):

1. Explicate order: "Unfolded: order structured in space and time; "what is."

2. Implicate order: "Enfolded" order; each region contains a total structure enfolded or latent within it; "what is to be."

ORDERING PRINCIPLES: Fundamental bases underlying the sequence, set, or pattern of an event or a behavior.

PRANA: Vital, life-giving force; breath.

SUPRAPHYSICAL: 1. Above. 2. Beyond; e.g., transcending the gross physical energies to the finer, vital energies.

TELERECEPTOR: A sensory organ that receives stimuli from a distance; for instance, the ear, which can hear sounds that have originated at a distance.

THYMUS: Lymphoid organ situated at the base of the breastbone, producing lymphocytes for the immune response.

UNIVERSAL FIELD: In principle, fields that extend throughout the measurable universe.

UNIVERSAL LIFE FIELD: Characterized by the ability to replenish the living energy called vitality.

VITAL SIGNS: Biological indicators characteristic of life; for example, respiration, pulse, and body temperature.

BIBLIOGRAPHY

Achterberg, J. and F. Lawlis. *Imagery Of Cancer: A Diagnostic Tool for the Process of Disease.* Champagne, IL: Institute for Personality and Ability Testing, 1978.

Ader, R. (ed.). *Psychoneuroimmunology.* New York: Academic Press. 1986.

Avalon, A. *The Serpent Power.* Madras: Ganesh & Co., 1964.

Beston, H. *The Outermost House.* New York: Holt, Rinehart and Winston, 1928.

Bohm, D. *Wholeness and Implicate Order.* London: Routledge and Kegan Paul, 1980.

Cannon, W. *The Wisdom of the Body.* London: Norton, 1932.

Capra, F. *The Tao of Physics.* Berkeley: Shambhala, 1975.

Cohen, K. "External Qi Healing: The Chinese Therapeutic Touch." *Qi - The Journal of Traditional Eastern Health and Fitness,* Summer 1993, pp.10-17.

Govinda, A. *Creative Meditation and Multi-Dimensional Consciousness.* Wheaton, IL: The Theosophical Publishing House, 1976.

Green, E. and A. Green. *Beyond Biofeedback.* New York: Delacourt Press, 1977.

Karagulla, S. and D. Kunz. *The Chakras and the Human Energy Field.* Wheaton, IL: Quest Books, 1989.

Krieger, D. "Therapeutic Touch: The Imprimatur of Nursing." *American Journal of Nursing,* Vol. 75, pp.784-787.

Krieger, D. *Therapeutic Touch: How to Use Your Hands to Help or to Heal.* Englewood Cliffs, NJ: Prentice-Hall Press, 1979.

Krieger, D. *Accepting Your Power To Heal: The Personal Practice of Therapeutic Touch.* Santa Fe: Bear & Co., 1993.

Krieger, D., E. Peper, and S. Ancoli. "Searching for Evidence of Physiological Change." *American Journal of Nursing,* Vol.79: pp.660-662.

Krippner, S. *Human Possibilities*. New York: Anchor Press, 1980.

Krippner, S. and A. Vollodo. *The Realms of Healing*. Millbrae, CA: Celestial Arts, 1976.

Kunz, D. "Compassion, Rootedness and Detachment: Their Role in Healing." In *Spiritual Aspects of the Healing Arts* (Dora Kunz, ed.). Wheaton, IL: Quest Books, 1985, pp.289-305.

Kunz, D. *The Personal Aura*. Wheaton, IL: Quest Books, 1991.

LeShan, L. *The Medium, The Mystic And The Physicist*. New York: Ballantine, 1974.

Maslow, A. *Toward A Psychology Of Being*. New York: Van Nostrand and Reinhold, 1968.

Mutwa, C. *My People*. Tribridge, Kent: Peach Hall Works, 1969.

Pelletier, K. *Mind The Healer, Mind The Slayer: An Holistic Approach to Preventing Stress Disorders*. New York: Dell Co., Inc., 1977.

Peters, D., P.J. Lewis, L. Chaitow, C. Watson. "Clinical Forum: Chronic Fatigue." *Complementary Therapies in Medicine,* January 1996, Vol. 4, #1, pp. 31-36.

Pribram, K. "Problems Concerning the Structure of Consciousness." In *Consciousness And The Brain* (G.G. Globus et al, eds.). New York: Plenum, 1976.

Sheldrake, R. *A New Science Of Life: The Hypothesis of Formative Causation*. London: Blond, 1981.

Schatz, A. and K. Carlson. "The Integration of Swedish Massage and Therapeutic Touch." *Massage and Bodyworks,* Spring 1995, pp.51-55.

Simonton, O., S. Simonton and J. Creighton. *Getting Well Again*. Los Angeles: Jeremy Tarcher, 1978.

Tart, C. *States of Consciousness*. New York: EP Dutton, 1975.

Tart, C. *Open Mind, Discriminating Mind*. San Francisco: Harper & Row, 1989.

Weber, R. *Dialogues with Scientists and Saints*. London: Routledge and Kegan Paul, 1986.

Wilber, K. *The Atman Project: A Transpersonal View of Human Development*. Wheaton, IL: Theosophical Publishing House, 1980.

INDEX

ABOUT THE AUTHOR

Dr. Krieger's life has been called a paradox: She has lived simultaneously in two worlds, and each world has bestowed upon her many honors. In the world of academia, she is professor emerita, New York University, and has been at the leading edge of research, theory development, and the clinical implementation of healing practices as a humane professional intervention.

In 1972, together with her colleague Dora Kunz, Dr. Krieger developed Therapeutic Touch, a contemporary interpretation of several ancient healing practices. They specifically developed Therapeutic Touch as an extension of professional skills for persons in the health field. Since 1984, when research by Dr. Krieger demonstrated both its feasibility and safety, Therapeutic Touch has been adapted for all people—children and adolescents as well as adults. Therapeutic Touch has now been taught in more than one hundred colleges and universities in the United States and in seventy-five foreign countries. In the world of alternative and collaborative healing modes, Therapeutic Touch is an acknowledged pioneer, for it has been consistently taught in fully accredited college and university curricula since 1975, an historical first.

Dr. Krieger's personal life reflects the far-flung scope of her interests. Her hobbies include French intensive organic gardening, mountain climbing, wood carving, rock collecting, reading ancient petroglyphs, and rebuilding old stone fences. She supports life-affirmative activities such as the humane protection of all endangered flora and fauna (including human beings at risk), and world-level coordinated, sustainable agricultural practices.

BOOKS OF RELATED INTEREST

Accepting Your Power to Heal
The Personal Practice of Therapeutic Touch
by Dolores Krieger, Ph.D., R.N.

The Spiritual Dimension of Therapeutic Touch
by Dora Kunz with Dolores Krieger, Ph.D., R.N

Reiki for the Heart and Soul
The Reiki Principles as Spiritual Pathwork
by Amy Z. Rowland

Intuitive Reiki for Our Times
Essential Techniques for Enhancing Your Practice
by Amy Z. Rowland

Traditional Reiki for Our Times
Practical Methods for Personal and Planetary Healing
by Amy Z. Rowland

Healing Stones for the Vital Organs
83 Crystals with Traditional Chinese Medicine
by Michael Gienger and Wolfgang Maier

Vibrational Medicine
The #1 Handbook of Subtle-Energy Therapies
by Richard Gerber, M.D.

Inner Traditions • Bear & Company
P.O. Box 388
Rochester, VT 05767
1-800-246-8648
www.InnerTraditions.com

Or contact your local bookseller